Pediatric Advanced Life Support Study Guide

Barbara Aehlert, R.N.
Southwest EMS Education, Inc.
Glendale, Arizona

Illustrations (except ECGs and those otherwise noted) by Kimberly Battista
Photography (unless otherwise noted) by Vincent Knaus

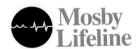

Mosby
Lifeline

St. Louis Baltimore Boston Carlsbad Chicago Naples New York Philadelphia Portland
London Madrid Mexico City Singapore Sydney Tokyo Toronto Wiesbaden

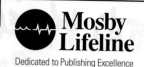

Mosby Lifeline
Dedicated to Publishing Excellence

Publisher: David T. Culverwell
Executive Editor: Richard A. Weimer
Developmental Editor: Julie Scardiglia
Editorial Assistant: Kay Beard
Book Design and Production: Cynthia Edmiston, Merrifield Graphics & Publishing Service, Inc.
Cover Illustration: Kimberly Battista

Mosby-Year Book, Inc.
11830 Westline Industrial Drive
St. Louis, MO 63146

PREFACE

The Pediatric Advanced Life Support Study Guide is designed for use as a workbook and reference to accompany the American Heart Association Pediatric Advanced Life Support text. Participants of the PALS Course predictably consist of physicians, nurses, respiratory therapists, prehospital providers and other allied health professionals whose background and exposure to the pediatric patient is significantly varied.

The Pediatric Advanced Life Support Study Guide follows the organization and format of the AHA material. This text is presented in outline form in an effort to provide the reader with a concise but comprehensive summary of the key points presented in the AHA text. The chapters in this text are consistent with those of the AHA text and provide instructional objectives followed by a review of the critical elements related to the subject. In addition, a pretest, posttest and quizzes with answers referenced to the 1994 AHA Pediatric Advanced Life Support text are provided for self-evaluation.

This text is designed to assist you in preparing for the Pediatric Advanced Life Support course, as an adjunct to the lectures and skills sessions provided during the course, and as a reference upon completion of the course. I hope you find this text of assistance and welcome your comments and suggestions.

Barbara Aehlert, R.N.

DEDICATION

For my editor,

Julie Scardiglia

whose commitment to excellence is evident in every project she undertakes.

I appreciate your advice, humor and wit. Your constant energy and
pleasant personality make each endeavor we undertake together a joy.
I am truly blessed to have been given the opportunity to work with you.

ACKNOWLEDGMENTS

I would like to thank:

Sean P. Newton, CEP and his daughter Brianna, and Nicholas and Cassandra Sivak, the models for the photographs used in this text. I sincerely appreciate your patience and willingness to assist us with this project.

Deby Campbell, RN, Nancy Kavic-Shaver, RN, Craig Laser, RN, and Cindy Gaspar-Rust, RN. A very special thanks to each of you. You have graciously shared your thoughts in stimulating discussions regarding the care of children.

David Beyda, M.D., David Tellez, M.D., and Paul Bakerman, M.D. of Phoenix Children's Hospital and Wendy Lucid, M.D. of Good Samaritan Regional Medical Center. I have learned from each of you and deeply respect your expertise in the management of ill and injured children.

Cathy J. June, BSN, RN, CEN, Lisa Magoteaux, RN, William Raynovich, Gary Rushworth, BS, RRT, and Laraine S. Yakowich, RN, BSN, the reviewers of the original manuscript. Your comments and suggestions are sincerely appreciated. I hope you will be pleased with the final product, which incorporates many of your suggestions.

Marcia Barry, RN, MSN, Mary Alice Witzel, RN, Suzanne Sawicki, and Julie McKinney, RN. You are always there when I need you.

Richard Weimer and David Culverwell of Mosby Lifeline for their support of this project and for allowing me the opportunity to continue working with Julie.

Cynthia Edmiston of Merrifield Graphics & Publishing Service, Inc., whose expertise and hours of preparation of the final product is sincerely appreciated. I enjoy working with you and appreciate your comments and suggestions.

Vincent Knaus, who patiently photographed the models and equipment for this text. I am pleased and honored to have had the opportunity to meet you. You have a wonderful personality and the quality of your work is exceptional.

Kimberly Battista, the text illustrator, whose talent is extraordinary. I am thankful we were able to work on another project together.

My husband Dean and daughters, Andrea and Sherri, who have been very patient with me while I completed this book.

CONTENTS

Pretest

1. Whenever possible, a pulse oximeter should be used during pediatric intubation.

   a. True
   b. False

2. List four medications that may be administered endotracheally.

   1. _____

   2. _____

   3. _____

   4. _____

3. Which of the following is NOT a desirable feature of a bag-valve device?

   a. a clear mask
   b. compressible, self-refilling bag
   c. pop-off (pressure release) valve
   d. availability in adult and pediatric sizes

4. Which of the following reflects proper management of sinus tachycardia?

   a. immediate defibrillation with 2 joules/kg
   b. administer 0.1 mg/kg of epinephrine IV push
   c. therapy should be directed at the underlying cause
   d. administer 0.02 mg/kg of atropine with a minimum dose of 1.0 mg

5. Calcium chloride is indicated for the treatment of:

   a. asystole
   b. hyperkalemia
   c. hyponatremia
   d. ventricular fibrillation

6. Local complications of intravascular access include:

   a. sepsis
   b. phlebitis
   c. air embolism
   d. pulmonary thromboembolism

7. The Seldinger technique:

   a. involves the insertion of a rigid spinal needle into the marrow of a lower extremity bone

b. helps minimize gastric distention and aspiration by means of pressure applied to the cricoid cartilage

c. allows the introduction of a large-bore over-the-needle-catheter into the chest to relieve a tension pneumothorax

d. allows the introduction of large catheters into the central venous circulation after initial venous entry with a small-gauge needle or over-the-needle-catheter

8. Rescue breaths are provided at a rate of approximately _____ for infants and children.

    a. 12 per minute

    b. 15 per minute

    c. 20 per minute

    d. 30 per minute

9. The recommended endotracheal dose of epinephrine is:

    a. 0.1 mg/kg of 1:1000 solution

    b. 0.01 mg/kg of 1:1000 solution

    c. 0.1 mg/kg of 1:10,000 solution

    d. 0.01 mg/kg of 1:10,000 solution

10. List five signs of respiratory failure.

    1. _____

    2. _____

    3. _____

    4. _____

    5. _____

11. The drug of choice for symptomatic supraventricular tachycardia (SVT) is:

    a. atropine

    b. lidocaine

    c. adenosine

    d. dobutamine

12. Transcutaneous pacing necessitates the use of two large adhesive-backed electrodes. If the child weighs less than _____, pediatric (small or medium) electrodes are recommended.

    a. 15 kilograms

    b. 25 kilograms

    c. 40 kilograms

    d. 50 kilograms

13. Retractions are:

    a. a high-pitched inspiratory sound associated with upper airway obstruction
    b. a bluish discoloration of the skin and mucous membranes from lack of oxygen
    c. a crackling sound caused by air entering the alveoli of the lungs that have a buildup of fluid
    d. a visible sinking-in of the soft tissues of the chest between the ribs associated with increased breathing effort

14. Which of the following is a crystalloid solution?

    a. dextran
    b. 5% albumin
    c. Ringer's lactate
    d. fresh frozen plasma

15. A 6 year old fell into a swimming pool and was pulled from the water by a neighbor. Rescue breathing has been initiated. Where should a pulse be checked in this child?

    a. apical
    b. carotid
    c. brachial
    d. femoral

16. The suggested endotracheal tube size for a six month old is:

    a. 2.5-3.0 mm I.D.
    b. 3.5-4.0 mm I.D.
    c. 4.5-5.0 mm I.D.
    d. 5.0-5.5 mm I.D.

17. Indications for defibrillation include:

    a. asystole
    b. symptomatic bradycardia
    c. supraventricular tachycardia
    d. pulseless ventricular tachycardia

18. The drug of choice for management of bradycardia with accompanying signs of severe cardiorespiratory compromise is:

    a. atropine
    b. epinephrine
    c. isoproterenol
    d. sodium bicarbonate

19. List four possible causes of pulseless electrical activity.

1. _____

2. _____

3. _____

4. _____

20. Cardiopulmonary arrest in children is usually due to profound hypoxemia and acidosis, often the result of a progressive deterioration in respiratory and circulatory function.

    a. true
    b. false

21. Indications for positive-pressure ventilation of the neonate include:

    1. Apnea or gasping respirations
    2. Heart rate < 100 beats per minute
    3. Respiratory rate of 40-60 breaths per minute
    4. Persistent cyanosis despite administration of 100% oxygen

    a. 1, 2, 3
    b. 1, 2, 4
    c. 1, 3, 4
    d. 2, 3, 4

22. A six year old child has suffered a cardiac arrest. The cardiac monitor displays ventricular fibrillation.

    a. Based on the child's age, you estimate his weight in kilograms to be

        _____.

    b. Proper energy levels for delivery of the initial "stacked" shock sequence to this patient would be _____ joules, _____ joules and _____ joules.

23. Respiratory failure is best described as:

    a. a clinical condition characterized by failure of the cardiovascular system to adequately perfuse vital organs
    b. a clinical condition characterized by deficits in oxygenation, ventilation and perfusion
    c. a clinical condition in which substantial cellular damage has been sustained due to poor oxygen delivery
    d. a clinical condition in which there is inadequate blood oxygenation and/or ventilation to meet the metabolic demands of body tissues

24. A six year old child in cardiac arrest has been intubated. Which of the following would indicate inadvertent esophageal intubation?

    a. subcutaneous emphysema
    b. external jugular vein distention
    c. gurgling sounds heard over the epigastrium
    d. breath sounds present on only one side of the chest

25. List the three categories of pediatric cardiac rhythms.

    1. _____

    2. _____

    3. _____

26. Respiratory acidosis in cardiopulmonary resuscitation is best managed by administering 100% oxygen and:

    a. glucose
    b. sodium bicarbonate
    c. increasing the rate of ventilations
    d. decreasing the rate of ventilations

27. A 6 month old male infant was last seen an hour ago when his mother put him down for a nap. The infant is pulseless and apneic. The cardiac monitor displays the rhythm below. CPR is begun and the infant is hyperventilated with 100% oxygen. An endotracheal tube is successfully placed. Breath sounds are present bilaterally and there is good chest rise. The first attempt at establishing venous access has proven unsuccessful. How should you proceed?

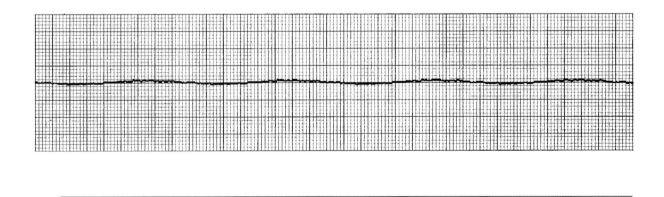

_____

_____

_____

28. Signs of early (compensated) shock include:
    1. Sinus tachycardia
    2. Hypotension
    3. Mottling or pallor
    4. Decreased strength of peripheral pulses
    5. Narrowed pulse pressure

    a. 1, 2
    b. 2, 3
    c. 1, 4, 5
    d. 3, 4, 5

29. Dobutamine is usually infused at a dose range of:
    a. 1-2 mg/kg/min
    b. 2-5 mg/kg/min
    c. 5-10 mcg/kg/min
    d. 10-20 mcg/kg/min

30. The standard paddle placement for pediatric defibrillation is:
    a. one paddle on the upper right chest below the clavicle, the other to the left of the left nipple in the anterior axillary line
    b. one paddle on the upper left chest below the clavicle, the other to the left of the left nipple in the anterior axillary line
    c. one paddle on the upper left chest below the clavicle, the other to the right of the right nipple in the anterior axillary line
    d. one paddle on the upper right chest below the clavicle, the other to the right of the right nipple in the anterior axillary line

31. Atropine is considered a Class I (definitely helpful) intervention in:
    a. ventricular fibrillation
    b. asystolic cardiac arrest
    c. supraventricular tachycardia
    d. symptomatic bradycardia with AV block

32. When sodium bicarbonate is used during cardiac arrest, 1 mEq/kg should be given as the initial dose and repeated every 5 minutes thereafter.
    a. true
    b. false

33. Which of the following objective signs of the Apgar score are the most important in rapidly assessing the need for resuscitation?

    1. Heart rate
    2. Respirations
    3. Muscle tone
    4. Reflex irritability
    5. Color

    a. 1, 4, 5
    b. 1, 2, 5
    c. 2, 3, 4
    d. 1, 3, 5

34. The recommended initial dose of bretylium is:

    a. 1 mg/kg
    b. 5 mg/kg
    c. 2.5-5 mg
    d. 5-10 mg

35. The term "unsynchronized countershock" is synonymous with defibrillation.

    a. true
    b. false

36. During cardiopulmonary resuscitation, the preferred site for vascular access in the pediatric patient is:

    a. a scalp vein
    b. the intraosseous route
    c. the external jugular or femoral vein
    d. the largest accessible vein that does not interrupt CPR

37. Synchronized countershock is indicated for the unstable patient with:

    a. asystole
    b. ventricular fibrillation
    c. pulseless electrical activity
    d. supraventricular tachycardia

38. Adenosine is the drug of choice for the treatment of:

    a. congestive heart failure
    b. supraventricular tachycardia
    c. calcium channel blocker overdose
    d. profound symptomatic bradycardia

39. Noninvasive (transcutaneous) pacing is indicated in:

    a. sinus tachycardia
    b. ventricular fibrillation
    c. symptomatic bradycardia refractory to BLS and ALS interventions
    d. symptomatic supraventricular tachycardia refractory to BLS and ALS interventions

40. The absolute refractory period:

    a. begins with the onset of the P wave and terminates with the end of the QRS complex
    b. begins with the onset of the QRS complex and terminates with the end of the T wave
    c. begins with the onset of the QRS complex and terminates at approximately the apex of the T wave
    d. begins with the onset of the P wave and terminates with the beginning of the QRS complex

41. A 3 year old female is the victim of a pedestrian motor vehicle accident. The patient was reportedly struck by a truck travelling at approximately 30 miles per hour. Examination reveals the airway to be clear with spinal precautions in place. The child is presently crying. Breath sounds are clear and equal bilaterally with good chest rise and a respiratory rate of 30 per minute. There is a superficial abrasion and ecchymosis noted on the right inferior chest. Pulses are palpable in all extremities though the hands and toes feel cool to the touch. Capillary refill is 3-4 seconds. The pulse rate is 150, blood pressure 86/70. The pupils are equal, round, and reactive to light. The abdomen appears distended and ecchymosis is noted to the left of the umbilicus. A superficial abrasion of the left knee is noted. The child moves all four extremities and recognizes her parents.

    What are the initial management priorities for this patient?

    _____

    _____

    _____

42. Describe two methods of evaluating heart rate in the neonate.

    1. _____

    2. _____

43. Select the incorrect statement regarding gastroenteritis.

    a. signs of dehydration precede shock
    b. gastroenteritis is most often a result of trauma
    c. rapid volume expansion may be necessary to prevent cardiovascular collapse
    d. the presence of gastrointestinal infection may result in shock due to hypovolemia

44. Renal and mesenteric vasodilation is thought to occur with stimulation of:

    a. dopaminergic receptors
    b. alpha-adrenergic receptors
    c. beta-1 adrenergic receptors
    d. beta-2 adrenergic receptors

45. Which of the following is considered a peripheral vein?

    a. femoral
    b. subclavian
    c. median basilic
    d. internal jugular

46. With an oxygen flow rate of 1-6 liters/minute, a nasal cannula can deliver an estimated oxygen concentration of:

    a. 17-21%
    b. 25-45%
    c. 45-60%
    d. 60-100%

47. Which of the following is used to suppress ventricular ectopy and raise the threshold for ventricular fibrillation?

    a. atropine
    b. lidocaine
    c. dopamine
    d. epinephrine

48. Oxygen should be administered as soon as possible to all pediatric patients with cardiac or respiratory arrest or suspected hypoxemia, regardless of cause.

    a. true
    b. false

49. Bronchodilation and vasodilation are effects that occur with stimulation of:

    a. beta-1 receptors
    b. beta-2 receptors
    c. alpha-1 receptors
    d. dopaminergic receptors

50. Which of the following reflects, in the order of most to least common frequency, the steps in neonatal resuscitation?

   1. Oxygen administration
   2. Chest compressions
   3. Administration of medications
   4. Drying, positioning, suction
   5. Establish effective ventilation

   a. 3, 1, 2, 4, 5
   b. 4, 1, 5, 2, 3
   c. 1, 2, 4, 5, 3
   d. 4, 3, 5, 1, 2

PRETEST ANSWERS

QUESTION	ANSWER	RATIONALE	STUDY GUIDE PAGE REFERENCE	PALS PAGE REFERENCE
1	A	Pulse oximeters monitor oxygen saturation and should be used whenever possible when intubating the pediatric patient.	101	4-15
2		Medications that may be administered may be remembered by "LEAN" or "LANE" - lidocaine, epinephrine, atropine and naloxone.	98	6-5, 6-6, 6-9
3	C	To properly ventilate patients in cardiac arrest, higher than usual airway pressures are often needed. Pop-off valves may prevent generation of sufficient peak airway pressure to overcome the increase in airway resistance.	93	4-12
4	C	Management of sinus tachycardia is directed at the underlying cause such as fever, pain, anxiety, hypoxia, hypovolemia.	156, 168	7-3
5	B	Calcium chloride is indicated for treatment of documented or suspected hypocalcemia, hyperkalemia, hypermagnesemia, and calcium channel blocker overdose.	144	6-11
6	B	Local complications of intravascular access include phlebitis, hematoma formation, cellulitis and thrombosis. Sepsis, air embolism and pulmonary thromboembolism are examples of systemic complications.	117	5-3

7	D	The Seldinger technique involves the use of a guidewire and allows the introduction of large catheters into the central venous circulation after initial venous entry with a small-gauge needle or over-the-needle-catheter.	116	5-7
8	C	Rescue breaths are provided for infants and children at a rate of approximately 20 breaths per minute.	39	3-10
9	A	Studies suggest that standard intravenous (IV) doses of epinephrine administered endotracheally (ET) produce serum levels approximately 10% or less than of an equivalent dose administered IV. The recommended endotracheal dose of epinephrine has been increased to 10 times the intravenous or intraosseous (IO) dose. The initial recommended IV/IO dose is 0.01 mg/kg of 1:10,000 solution in pulseless arrest. The ET dose is 0.1 mg/kg of 1:1000 solution.	141	6-15
10		Signs of respiratory failure include: diminished breath sounds, cyanosis, decreased level of consciousness or response to pain, poor skeletal muscle tone, inadequate respiratory rate, increased effort or chest excursion.	44, 52-53	2-2
11	C	The drug of choice for symptomatic supraventricular tachycardia is adenosine.	145	7-5
12	A	If the child weighs less than 15 kilograms, pediatric (small or medium) electrodes are recommended for use when initiating transcutaneous pacing.	166	7-11
13	D	Retractions are a visible sinking-in of the soft tissues of the chest between the ribs associated with increased breathing effort. (A) describes stridor. (B) describes cyanosis. (C) describes rales.	51	2-3

14	C	Ringer's lactate and normal saline are examples of crystalloid solutions. 5% albumin, fresh frozen plasma, Hetastarch and Dextran are colloid solutions.	114	6-1
15	B	The carotid pulse should be checked in the child over the age of 1 year.	26	3-7
16	B	The suggested endotracheal tube size for a 6 month old is 3.5 or 4.0 mm internal diameter (uncuffed).	106	4-15
17	D	Indications for defibrillation include pulseless ventricular tachycardia and ventricular fibrillation.	164	7-8
18	B	The drug of choice for bradycardia associated with signs of severe cardiorespiratory compromise is epinephrine.	167	7-7
19		Causes of pulseless electrical activity may be remembered by PATH(x3): Pneumothorax (tension), Acidosis (severe), Tamponade (cardiac), Hypoxemia (severe), Hypovolemia (severe), Hypothermia (profound)	161, 170	7-9
20	A	Cardiopulmonary arrest in children is usually due to profound hypoxemia and acidosis, often the result of a progressive deterioration in respiratory and circulatory function. Cardiac arrest in the adult is primarily cardiac in origin.	19, 42	2-1
21	B	Indications for positive-pressure ventilation in the neonate include: apnea or gasping respirations, heart rate < 100 beats/minute or persistent central cyanosis despite administration of 100% oxygen.	194	9-5

22		a. The patient's weight in kilograms may be estimated by using the formula 8 + (years x 2). Thus, this child's estimated kilogram weight would be 20 kg. b. "Stacked" shocks should be delivered with 2 joules/kg initially and repeated, if necessary, with 4 joules/kg and 4 joules/kg. Thus, energy settings for this child would be 40 joules, 80 joules and 80 joules.	169	7-8, 7-9
23	D	Respiratory failure is a clinical condition in which there is inadequate blood oxygenation and/or ventilation to meet the metabolic demands of body tissues. (A) describes shock. (B) describes cardiopulmonary failure and (C) describes multiple-organ system failure.	43	2-1
24	C	Absence of chest rise and gurgling heard over the epigastrium indicate misplacement of the endotracheal tube into the esophagus.	104-105	4-17
25		The three categories of pediatric cardiac rhythms are: 1. Fast rhythms 2. Slow rhythms 3. Disorganized, absent or collapse rhythms	156-160	7-3
26	C	Respiratory acidosis in cardio-pulmonary arrest is best treated by administration of 100% oxygen and increasing the rate of ventilation.	144	6-3

27		The rhythm displayed is asystole. Confirm the rhythm in another lead. Since the endotracheal tube is in place and tube position has been confirmed, administer epinephrine 0.1 mg/kg of 1:1000 solution (0.1 ml/kg) endotracheally. Epinephrine may be repeated in 3-5 minutes. If vascular access has not been obtained (either IV or IO), administer a second dose of epinephrine endotracheally. Reevaluate the adequacy of ventilation and chest compressions frequently.	160	7-9
28	C	Signs of early (compensated) shock include sinus tachycardia, decreased strength of peripheral pulses, narrowed pulse pressure. Mottling or pallor and hypotension are signs of late (decompensated) shock.	61	2-4
29	C	Dobutamine is usually begun at 5-10 mL per hour, which delivers 5-10 mcg/kg/min when mixed as follows: 6 mg dobutamine x child's body weight in kilograms. This is the mg dose added to sufficient diluent to create a total volume of 100 mL.	149	6-13, 6-16
30	A	The standard paddle placement for pediatric defibrillation is one paddle on the upper right chest below the clavicle, the other to the left of the left nipple in the anterior axillary line.	162	7-10
31	D	Atropine is considered a Class I (definitely helpful) intervention in symptomatic bradycardia with AV block (an uncommon event) and vagally mediated bradycardia during intubation attempts. Atropine is considered a Class IIb (possibly helpful) intervention in asystole and is not indicated in the management of ventricular fibrillation.	146	6-8, 6-9

32	B	When used, 1 mEq/kg should be administered as the initial dose of sodium bicarbonate and subsequent doses based on blood gas analysis. If blood gas results are unavailable, subsequent doses of bicarbonate may be considered after every 10 minutes of cardiac arrest.	144	6-8, 6-15
33	B	The need for resuscitation can be more rapidly assessed by evaluating the heart rate, respiratory activity and color than by the total Apgar score.	191-192	9-5
34	B	The recommended dose of bretylium is 5 mg/kg rapid IV infusion in ventricular fibrillation. This dose may be increased to 10 mg/kg if VF persists after defibrillation. If administered for refractory or recurrent ventricular tachycardia (conscious patient), the recommended dose is 5 mg/kg infused over 8-10 minutes to reduce the likelihood of nausea and vomiting.	147	6-15, 7-9
35	A	Countershock and cardioversion are general terms. Unsynchronized countershock (or unsynchronized cardioversion) is synonymous with defibrillation and refers to the random delivery of energy during the cardiac cycle.	161	7-8
36	D	If no IV exists prior to a cardiopulmonary arrest, the preferred access site is the largest, most easily accessible vein that does not interrupt CPR.	114	5-1
37	D	Synchronized countershock (cardioversion) is indicated for the unstable patient with SVT, VT with a pulse, atrial fibrillation, or atrial flutter. Defibrillation (unsynchronized countershock) is indicated for ventricular fibrillation. Countershock is not indicated in asystole or pulseless electrical activity.	165	7-4

38	B	Adenosine is the drug of choice for management of symptomatic supraventricular tachycardia.	145	7-5
39	C	Noninvasive (transcutaneous) pacing is indicated in cases of profound symptomatic bradycardia refractory to BLS and ALS interventions.	166	7-11
40	C	The absolute refractory period begins with the onset of the QRS complex and terminates at approximately the apex of the T wave. During this period, the cell cannot propagate or conduct an impulse.	153	N/A
41		The patient is presenting with signs and symptoms of early shock as evidenced by delayed capillary refill, cool extremities, diminished pulse pressure and a normal blood pressure. Initial management priorities include: deliver 100% oxygen, place the child on a cardiorespiratory monitor, obtain vascular access and administer a 20 ml/kg crystalloid fluid bolus (in < 20 minutes), reevaluate ABCs.	61-62	2-4, 6-2
42		Heart rate in the neonate may be evaluated by listening to the apical beat with a stethoscope, feeling the pulse by lightly grasping the base of the umbilical cord, monitoring with a cardiotachometer, or by palpating the brachial or femoral pulse.	191	9-4
43	B	Gastroenteritis is an inflammation of the stomach and intestines. It is usually caused by a virus but may be caused by a viral infection. Hypovolemia due to fluid loss secondary to diarrhea and vomiting may cause shock in infants and children. Signs of dehydration precede signs of shock. Rapid volume expansion may be needed to prevent cardiovascular collapse.	68	2-8

44	A	Renal and mesenteric vasodilation is thought to occur with stimulation of dopaminergic receptors.	138	6-12
45	C	The median basilic vein of the forearm is a peripheral vein. The femoral, subclavian and internal jugular are central veins.	118	5-4, 5-7
46	B	At 1-6 liters per minute of oxygen flow, a nasal cannula can deliver an oxygen concentration of approximately 25-45%.	84	N/A
47	B	Lidocaine is used to suppress ventricular ectopy and raise the ventricular fibrillation threshold.	147	
48	A	Oxygen should be administered as soon as possible to all patients (adult or pediatric) with cardiac or respiratory arrest or suspected hypoxemia, regardless of cause.	83	6-14
49	B	Bronchodilation and vasodilation are effects of beta-2 receptor stimulation.	138	N/A
50	B	The preferred sequence of events in neonatal resuscitation: 1. Drying, warming, positioning, suction, tactile stimulation 2. Oxygen administration 3. Establish effective ventilation • Bag valve mask • Endotracheal intubation 4. Chest compressions 5. Medications	188	9-1

Basic Life Support

OBJECTIVES

Upon completion of this chapter, you will be able to:

1. Name the common causes of cardiopulmonary arrest in infancy.
2. List the most common childhood injuries.
3. Describe the head-tilt/chin-lift and jaw-thrust methods for opening the airway.
4. Describe the preferred method of opening the airway in cases of suspected cervical spine injury.
5. State the proper ventilation and compression rates for infants and children when performing cardiopulmonary resuscitation.
6. Describe the differences in proper hand position when performing external chest compressions in infants and children.
7. Name the signs and symptoms of airway obstruction.
8. Describe the procedures used to relieve foreign body airway obstruction in infants and children.

EPIDEMIOLOGY OF CARDIOPULMONARY ARREST

Predisposing Factors

1. Ventricular fibrillation has been reported in only 10%-15% of children less than 10 years of age who experienced pulseless arrest outside of the hospital. VT or VF is more likely to be observed in children 10 years of age or older, submersion victims, children with congenital heart disease, and children who arrest in the hospital.[1]
2. Asystolic cardiac arrest in infants and children is usually the result of progressive hypoxemia and acidosis secondary to respiratory or circulatory failure
3. Pediatric cardiopulmonary arrest occurs most commonly under 1 year of age and during the teenage years
   a. During infancy, the most common causes of arrest include: sepsis, submersion, neurological disease, respiratory diseases, sudden infant death syndrome (SIDS), and airway obstruction (including foreign body aspiration)
   b. After 1 year of age, injuries are the leading cause of cardiopulmonary arrest in the pediatric patient

| Outcome | 1. Survival from asystolic cardiac arrest is estimated at less than 10%
    • Many of those who are resuscitated suffer permanent neurological damage
2. Survival rates from prompt resuscitation of children suffering respiratory arrest alone are nearly 50% |

INJURY PREVENTION

Most Common Childhood Injuries[2]	1. Motor vehicle passenger injuries 2. Pedestrian injuries 3. Bicycle injuries 4. Submersion 5. Burns 6. Firearm injuries
Motor Vehicle Injuries	Nearly 1/2 of all pediatric injuries and deaths are associated with motor-vehicle related trauma Contributing factors: 1. Failure to use proper passenger restraints 2. Inexperienced adolescent drivers 3. Alcohol abuse • Approximately 50% of adolescent motor vehicle fatalities involve alcohol[3]
Pedestrian Injuries	Leading cause of death among children 5 to 9 years of age • Child typically bolts out into the street
Bicycle Injuries	1. Head injuries are the cause of most bicycle-related morbidity and mortality 2. Bicycle-related trauma is the leading cause of severe pediatric closed-head injuries[4]
Submersion	1. Drowning is a significant cause of death and disability in children under 4 years of age 2. Leading cause of death in children under the age of 4 in several states

Burns	1. Approximately 80% of fire and burn-related deaths result from house fires
	a. Most fire-related deaths occur in private residences
	b. Many of these residences do not have working smoke detectors
	2. Children up to the age of 4 years are most likely to be affected by:
	a. Smoke inhalation
	b. Scalds
	c. Contact and electric burns
Firearm Injuries	1. The leading cause of death among African-American adolescents and young adults is firearm homicide
	2. The U.S. has a higher firearm-related homicide rate among young males than any industrialized nation, four times more than that of any other country.

THE ABCs OF CPR

AIRWAY

Assessment	1. Determine unresponsiveness or respiratory difficulty
	a. Quickly assess the presence or extent of any injury or respiratory difficulty and determine whether the child is conscious
	• Determine the level of responsiveness by tapping the child and speaking loudly
	• If head or neck trauma is suspected, do not shake the child to avoid spinal injury
	b. If the child is unresponsive but breathing, activate the EMS system to facilitate transport of the child as rapidly as possible to an advanced life support (ALS) facility
	c. The child with respiratory distress should be allowed to remain in the position he/she finds most comfortable in order to maintain patency of the partially obstructed airway

2. Call for help

    a. If alone, perform basic life support for one minute **before** activating the EMS system

        •   Respiratory arrest is more common than cardiac arrest in the pediatric patient

        •   May prevent progression of respiratory arrest to cardio-respiratory arrest

    b. If a second rescuer is present, the second rescuer should activate the EMS system

3. Position the victim

    a. Essential for the victim to be supine on a firm, flat surface for CPR to be effective

    b. Maintain manual in-line cervical spine stabilization if cervical spine injury is suspected

        •   Avoid extension, flexion and rotation of the neck

    c. When moving the child, the head and body must be held and turned as a unit with the head and neck firmly supported so the head does not roll, twist or tilt backward or forward

4. Open the airway

    a. Muscle relaxation and posterior displacement of the tongue causes airway obstruction in the unconscious victim

    b. If the victim is unconscious and trauma is **not** suspected, open the airway using the head-tilt/chin-lift maneuver

    c. If the victim is unconscious and trauma **IS** suspected, open the airway using the jaw-thrust maneuver **without head-tilt** when the cervical spine is completely immobilized

    d. If the child is conscious but demonstrating signs of respiratory difficulty, do not waste time attempting to open the airway - transport to an advanced life support facility as quickly as possible.

Head-Tilt/Chin-Lift

Procedure

1. Place the hand closest to the child's head on the forehead and tilt the head gently back into a neutral or slightly extended position

2. Place the fingers, but not the thumb, of the other hand under the bony part of the lower jaw at the chin- lift upward and outward

   • Avoid using the mouth or pushing on the soft tissues under the chin (doing so may obstruct the airway)

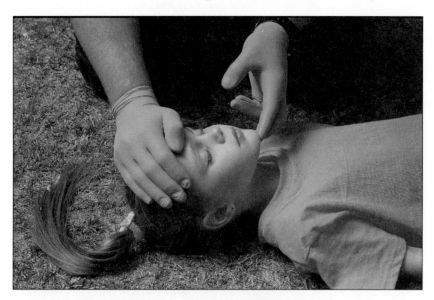

Figure 1-1. Head-tilt/chin-lift.

Jaw Thrust

Procedure

1. Place 2-3 fingers under each side of the lower jaw at its angle and lift the jaw upward and outward

2. The rescuer's elbows may rest on the surface on which the victim is lying

3. If trauma is not suspected and the jaw-thrust alone does not open the airway, the jaw-thrust may be accompanied by a slight head-tilt.

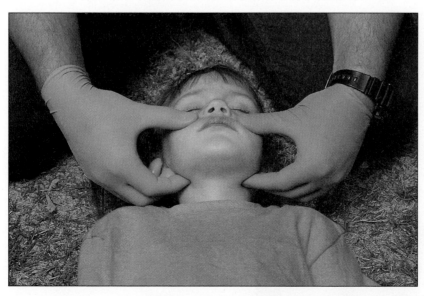

Figure 1-2. Jaw-thrust.

BREATHING

Assessment

Determine if the child is breathing:

1. **LOOK** for rise and fall of the chest and abdomen
2. **LISTEN** for exhaled air
3. **FEEL** for exhaled air flow
   - If the child is breathing, maintain a patent airway
   - If the child is not breathing, begin rescue breathing while maintaining a patent airway with a chin-lift or jaw-thrust

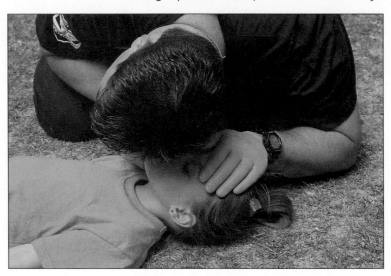

Figure 1-3. Look, listen and feel for breathing.

Rescue Breathing

Ventilation is the most important rescue maneuver for a nonbreathing infant or child.

Infant (less than 1 year of age)

Make a seal with the victim's mouth and nose

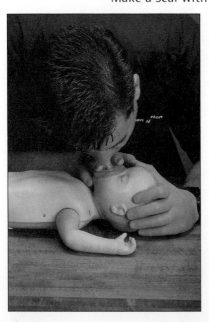

Figure 1-4. Rescue breathing for the infant.

Large infant or child (1-8 years of age)

Make a seal with the victim's mouth and pinch the victim's nose with the thumb and forefingers of the hand that is maintaining a head-tilt

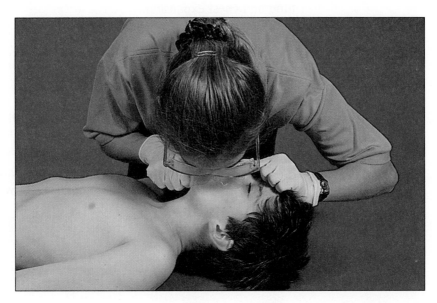

Figure 1-5.   Rescue breathing for the child. (From Stoy/Center for Emergency Medicine: Mosby's EMT-Basic Textbook, St. Louis, 1996, Mosby–Year Book.

Rescue breathing should be provided with a mask equipped with a one-way valve or similar device. Personal protective equipment should always be readily available, including masks with one-way valves for ventilating pediatric patients.

Deliver two slow breaths (1-1$\frac{1}{2}$ seconds per breath), pausing after the first breath.

1.   Allows the rescuer to take a breath to maximize oxygen content and minimize carbon dioxide concentration in delivered breaths.

  •   Failing to do so will result in rescue breaths low in oxygen and high in carbon dioxide

2.   By delivering breaths slowly, an effective tidal volume will be delivered at the lowest possible pressure, minimizing gastric distention

  •   Rapid rescue breathing may cause gastric distention

  •   Excessive gastric distention may inhibit rescue breathing by elevating the diaphragm and reducing lung volume

1. The volume of air delivered should be sufficient to cause gentle chest rise.

   • If the child's chest does not rise during rescue breathing, ventilation is not effective. Slow delivery of breaths will allow an adequate volume of air to be delivered and ensure effective lung and chest expansion.[5]

2. The airway is clear if air enters freely and the chest rises.

3. If the chest does not rise:

   a. The airway is obstructed

   b. More breath volume or pressure is needed

      • Most common cause of obstruction is improper opening of the airway. Readjust the head-tilt/chin-lift position, ensure the mouth is open and reattempt to ventilate

      • Suspect foreign body obstruction if the airway remains obstructed despite attempts to open the airway

CIRCULATION

Pulse Check

1. In children over the age of 1 year, the most accessible central artery is the carotid (neck)

2. In infants (less than 1 year of age), palpation of the brachial or femoral arteries are recommended because palpation of the carotid artery in a short, chubby neck is often difficult

   • The apical pulse is not used to determine the presence of a pulse because a precordial impulse (not a pulse) may not be felt despite the presence of strong central pulses and satisfactory cardiac function

Pulse Check - Infant

Procedure

1. Place the thumb on the outside of the victim's arm and the index and middle fingers on the inside of the upper arm, between the elbow and the shoulder

2. Press gently until the brachial pulse is felt

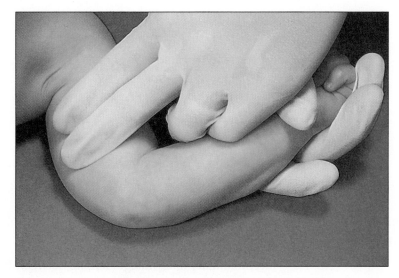

Figure 1-6. Locating the brachial pulse. (From Stoy/Center for
Emergency Medicine: Mosby's EMT-Basic Textbook,
St. Louis 1996, Mosby–Year Book.)

Pulse Check - Child

Procedure

1. Locate the child's Adam's apple with 2-3 fingers of one hand while maintaining a head-tilt with the other hand on the forehead.

2. Slide the fingers into the groove between the trachea and the sternocleidomastoid muscles and gently palpate the carotid artery (on the side closest to the rescuer)

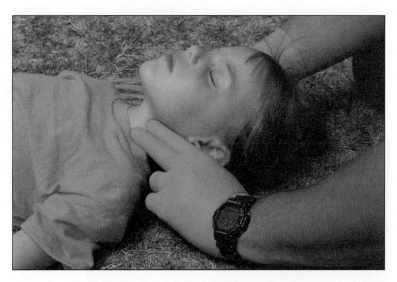

Figure 1-7. Locating the carotid pulse.

1. If a pulse is present but breathing is absent:

   a. Continue ventilation at a rate of 20 breaths per minute (one every 3 seconds) until breathing resumes

   b. After delivering 20 breaths, activate the EMS system

2. If a pulse is not present, begin chest compressions and coordinate with ventilation

Chest Compressions -
Indications

1. Asystole
2. Other non-perfusing rhythms
   a. Pulseless ventricular tachycardia
   b. Ventricular fibrillation

The child must be positioned on a hard surface in a horizontal, supine position

- The rescuer's hand or forearm with the palm supporting the back can be the hard surface for infant resuscitation

Chest Compressions - Infant
(less than 1 year of age)

1. Locate landmarks
   a. Lower 1/3 of the sternum
   b. Intermammary line - imaginary line between the nipples over the sternum
   c. Place the index finger of the hand farthest from the infant's head just below the intermammary line. Place the middle and ring fingers next to the index finger on the sternum. Perform chest compressions with the middle and ring fingers approximately one finger's breadth below the intermammary line.
2. Perform chest compressions
   a. Compress the sternum approximately 1/3 to 1/2 the depth of the chest (approximately 1/2 to 1 inch) at a rate of at least 100 times per minute
   b. The number of compressions will actually be at least 80 per minute due to pauses for ventilation
   c. Release pressure at the end of each compression without removing the fingers from the chest
   d. The rhythm should allow equal time for compression and relaxation

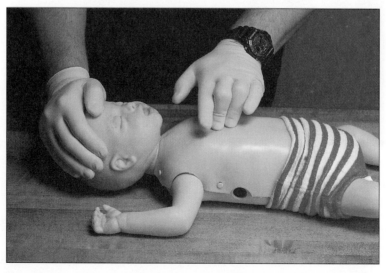

Figure 1-8. Locating finger position for infant chest compression.

Chest Compressions - Child
(1 to 8 years of age)

1. Locate landmarks

   a. On the side of the chest next to the rescuer, trace the lower margin of the child's rib cage using the middle and index fingers of the hand nearer the child's feet

   b. Place the middle finger in the notch where the ribs and sternum meet and place the index finger next to the middle finger

   c. Place the heel of the same hand next to where the index finger was located, with the long axis of the heel parallel to that of the sternum. The heel of the hand should remain in contact with the sternum while the fingers are held up off the ribs

2. Perform chest compressions

   a. Compress the sternum approximately 1/3 to 1/2 the depth of the chest (approximately 1 to 1 1/2 inches) at a rate of 100 times per minute

   b. The number of compressions will actually be approximately 80 per minute due to pauses for ventilation

   c. Release pressure at the end of each compression without removing the hand from the chest

   d. The rhythm should allow equal time for compression and relaxation

   e. Chest compressions should be delivered as in adult CPR if the child is large or older than the age of 8 years.

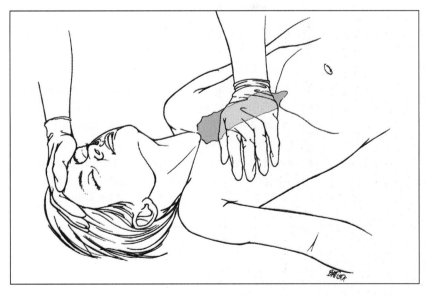

Figure 1-9. Locating hand position for child chest compression.

COORDINATION OF CHEST COMPRESSIONS AND RESCUE BREATHING

1. External chest compressions must be accompanied by ventilation
2. Allow a pause of 1 to $1\frac{1}{2}$ seconds at the end of every 5th compression for a ventilation
3. The compression to ventilation ratio is 5:1 for the infant and child (one and two rescuers). Two rescuer technique should only be used by healthcare providers.
4. Reassess for spontaneous breathing and pulse after 20 cycles of compressions and ventilation (approximately 1 minute) and every few minutes thereafter.

Single-Rescuer CPR - Infant

1. Maintain a patent airway with a head-tilt using the hand that is not performing chest compressions
   - Helps to lessen the time required to open the airway after every 5th compression, permitting delivery of an adequate number of chest compressions and ventilation per minute

2. Assure the chest expands adequately with each rescue breath delivered
   - After providing a rescue breath, return the hand to the chest to resume chest compressions

Single-Rescuer CPR - Child

1. The head-tilt maneuver alone is often insufficient to maintain a patent airway in the child, therefore both hands are used to perform the head-tilt/chin-lift maneuver with **each** ventilation.
2. After performing the head-tilt/chin-lift maneuver, the hand performing chest compressions is moved back to the chest. **Visualize** the chest and place the hand in the approximate location used previously for chest compressions.
   - Time is not taken to go through the full procedure to locate landmarks after each ventilation since the total number of chest compressions delivered would be significantly reduced.

ACTIVATING THE EMS SYSTEM

1. If the rescuer is alone, activate the EMS system after performing rescue efforts for approximately 1 minute (in cardiopulmonary arrest, 20 cycles of rescue breaths and chest compressions)

2. If the victim resumes spontaneous breathing and head and neck trauma is not suspected, turn the victim to the side (recovery position) before leaving the victim to activate the EMS system.

3. If a second rescuer is present or arrives while rescue efforts are in progress, one rescuer should activate the EMS system by calling the local emergency number (911 in many communities).

4. If trauma is not suspected and the victim is small, the child may be carried (while carefully supporting the head and neck) to a telephone while performing CPR to activate the EMS system.

5. If the rescuer is alone and unable to activate the EMS system, continue CPR until help arrives or the rescuer becomes too fatigued to continue rescue efforts.

Information for the EMS Dispatcher

The EMS dispatcher should be provided the following information:

1. Location of the emergency
    *   Include the address and names of streets or landmarks
2. Telephone number from which the call is being made
3. What happened (drowning, choking victim, auto accident)
4. Number of victims
5. Condition of the victim(s)
6. Nature of the aid being given
7. Any other information requested

NOTE: The caller should be the last to hang up.

FOREIGN-BODY AIRWAY OBSTRUCTION

Statistics	1. More than 90% of deaths from foreign-body aspiration in the pediatric age group occur in children younger than 5 years of age
	2. 65% of the victims are infants
Commonly Aspirated Materials	1. Toys
	• Consumer product safety standards regulating the minimum size of toys and toy parts has helped to decrease the incidence of foreign-body aspiration
	2. Small objects
	3. Foods
	• Grapes
	• Round candies
	• Nuts
	• Hot dogs
Signs and Symptoms of Airway Obstruction	1. Foreign-body airway obstruction should be suspected in infants and children with a *sudden* onset of respiratory distress associated with coughing, gagging, stridor or wheezing.
	2. Airway obstruction may also be caused by infections that cause swelling of the airway such as epiglottitis or croup. Infection should be suspected if the child has a fever, particularly if accompanied by:
	a. Drooling
	b. Lethargy
	c. Limpness
	d. Congestion
	e. Hoarseness[6]

MANAGING THE OBSTRUCTED AIRWAY

Attempt to Clear the Airway when:	1. Foreign-body aspiration is witnessed or strongly suspected.
	a. Encourage coughing and breathing efforts as long as the cough is forceful
	b. Attempt to relieve the obstruction only if:
	• The cough is or becomes ineffective (loss of sound)
	• There is increased respiratory difficulty accompanied by stridor
	• Or the victim becomes unconscious
	2. The airway remains obstructed (no chest rise) during attempts to provide rescue breathing to the unconscious, nonbreathing child.

Infant - Back Blows/
Chest Thrusts

A combination of back blows and chest thrusts are recommended for management of foreign-body airway obstruction in the infant.

- The Heimlich maneuver is not recommended in the infant as it is thought that abdominal thrusts may cause potentially fatal laceration of the relatively large and unprotected liver[7]

Procedure

1. Place the infant face down with his/her head lower than the trunk, over the rescuer's forearm.

2. Using the heel of one hand, deliver up to 5 back blows forcefully between the shoulder blades.

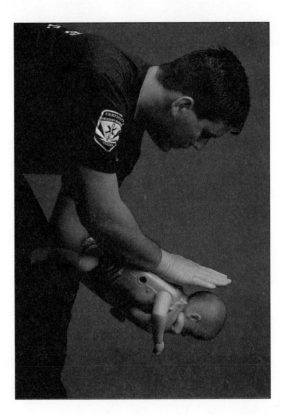

Figure 1-10. Delivering back blows to relieve foreign-body airway obstruction in the infant.

3. After delivering the back blows, the free hand should be used to hold the infant's head and support the back. The other hand is used to support the head, jaw and chest. The infant should be sandwiched between the rescuer's hands/arms and turned on his/her back, with the head lower than the trunk. Up to 5 chest thrusts should be delivered in the lower 1/3 of the sternum, approximately one finger's breadth below the intermammary line.

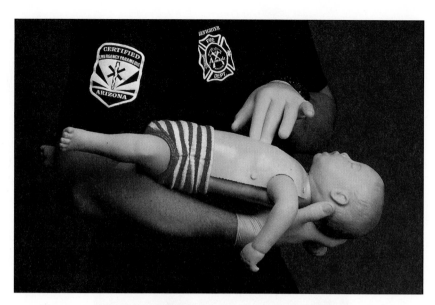

Figure 1-11. Delivering chest-thrusts to relieve foreign-body
airway obstruction in the infant.

Tongue-jaw lift - opening
of the victim's mouth by
grasping the tongue and
lower jaw between the
thumb and finger and lifting

4.   Perform a tongue-jaw lift and remove the foreign body if it is
visualized.

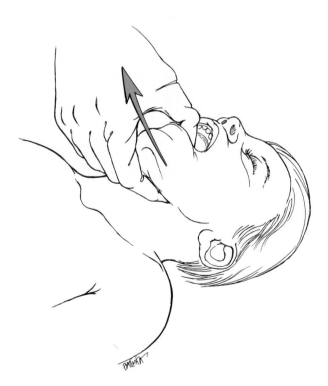

Figure 1-12. The tongue-jaw lift.

5. Open the airway and attempt to ventilate.
    a. If the chest does not rise, reposition the head and reattempt to ventilate.
    b. If the airway remains obstructed (absence of chest rise), repeat back blows, chest thrusts and attempts to ventilate until the object is removed and rescue breathing is effective.
6. When the obstruction is removed, assess for breathing.
    a. If breathing is present, place the infant on his/her side and continue to assess breathing and pulse while maintaining an open airway.
    b. If breathing is absent but a pulse is present, deliver 1 breath every 3 seconds (20 breaths per minute) and monitor the pulse.

Child - Heimlich Maneuver

The Heimlich maneuver is a series of subdiaphragmatic abdominal thrusts and is recommended for management of foreign-body airway obstruction in the child.

-   Subdiaphragmatic abdominal thrusts increase intrathoracic pressure, creating an artificial cough, forcing air and the foreign body out of the airway

Conscious Child Standing or Sitting

Procedure

1. The rescuer makes a fist by grasping his/her thumb with the right hand and stands behind the child, placing the thumbside of the fist against the child's abdomen in the midline slightly above the umbilicus.
2. The fist is grasped with the rescuer's other hand and a series of up to 5 quick, upward thrusts is delivered.
3. Continue until the foreign-body is expelled or the child becomes unconscious.
4. If the child becomes unconscious, place the child in a supine position and use the tongue-jaw lift to visualize the airway. If the foreign body is seen, remove it. **(No blind finger sweeps.)** Open the airway with a head-tilt/chin-lift or head-tilt/jaw-thrust. Attempt to ventilate. If the chest does not rise, reposition the head and reattempt to ventilate. If the airway remains obstructed (absence of chest rise), repeat the Heimlich maneuver and attempts to ventilate until the object is removed and rescue breathing is effective.

5. When the obstruction is removed, assess for breathing.

    a. If breathing is present, place the child on his/her side and continue to assess breathing and pulse while maintaining an open airway.

    b. If breathing is absent but a pulse is present, deliver 1 breath every 3 seconds (20 breaths per minute) and monitor the pulse.

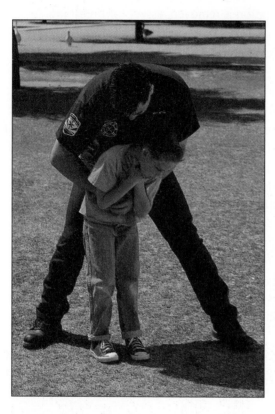

Figure 1-13. Performing the Heimlich maneuver on the conscious child standing.

Conscious or Unconscious Child Lying Down

1. Place the child in a supine position.

2. Open the airway and assess breathing.

3. Attempt to ventilate. If unsuccessful, reposition the head and reattempt to ventilate.

4. If the airway remains obstructed, kneel beside the child or straddle the child's hips. Place the heel of one hand on the child's abdomen in the midline slightly above the umbilicus. Place the other hand on top of the first.

5. Deliver up to 5 abdominal thrusts, pressing both hands into the abdomen with quick, upward thrusts directed toward the midline.

6. If the foreign-body is seen, remove it. **(No blind finger sweeps.)** Open the airway with a head-tilt/chin-lift or head-tilt/jaw-thrust. Attempt to ventilate. If the chest does not rise, reposition the head and reattempt to ventilate. If the airway remains obstructed (absence of chest rise), repeat the abdominal thrusts and attempts to ventilate until the object is removed and rescue breathing is effective.

7. When the obstruction is removed, assess for breathing.

   a. If breathing is present, place the child on his/her side and continue to assess breathing and pulse while maintaining an open airway.

   b. If breathing is absent but a pulse is present, deliver 1 breath every 3 seconds (20 breaths per minute) and monitor the pulse.

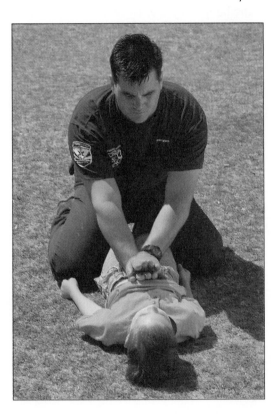

Figure 1-14. Performing the Heimlich maneuver on the conscious or unconscious child lying down.

CONSIDERATIONS IN PEDIATRIC TRAUMA

Anatomical Considerations

The pediatric trauma victim is predisposed to airway obstruction because:

1. The child's relatively large head causes slight flexion of the neck when the child is placed in a supine position on a flat surface.

2. The large tongue occludes the airway and the narrow trachea is susceptible to occlusion with vomitus or blood.

3. The preschool child may have loose teeth which are easily dislodged and may obstruct the airway.

4. Loss of pharyngeal tone and the gag reflex in the obtunded or comatose child.[8]

Suspected Head or Neck Injury

1. If head or neck injury is suspected, the cervical spine should be immobilized with the head in a neutral position and the airway opened using the jaw-thrust maneuver without head-tilt.

   - The head-tilt/chin-lift maneuver may worsen existing cervical spine injury and is contraindicated in cases of suspected head or neck injury.

2. The airway should ideally be managed with two rescuers - one to open the airway with the jaw-thrust maneuver while the other maintains manual in-line stabilization of the cervical spine (combined jaw-thrust and spinal stabilization maneuver).

   - "Traction on or movement of the neck must be avoided because it may result in conversion of a partial to a complete spinal cord injury."[9]

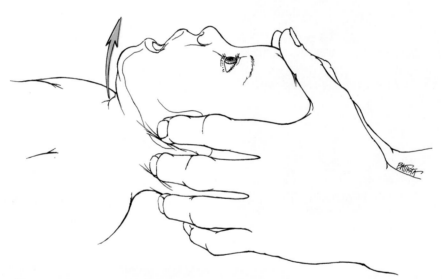

Figure 1-15. Combined jaw-thrust and spinal stabilization maneuver.

Table 1-1. Differences in Basic Life Support Interventions in Infants, Children and Adults

DIFFERENCES IN BASIC LIFE SUPPORT INTERVENTIONS IN INFANTS, CHILDREN AND ADULTS

	INFANT	CHILD	ADULT
Age	Under 1 year	1 to 8 years	Older than 8 years
Ventilation Rate	Initially 2 slow breaths (1-1 1/2 seconds per breath) Subsequently 1 breath every 3 seconds (20 breaths/minute)	Initially 2 slow breaths (1-1 1/2 seconds per breath) Subsequently 1 breath every 3 seconds (20 breaths/minute)	Initially 2 slow breaths (1 1/2-2 seconds per breath) Subsequently 1 breath every 5 seconds (12 breaths/minute)
Pulse Check	Brachial/femoral	Carotid	Carotid
Compression With	2 or 3 fingers	Heel of one hand	Heels of both hands
Depth	1/3 to 1/2 the depth of the chest (approximately 1/2 to 1 inch)	1/3 to 1/2 the depth of the chest (approximately 1 to 1-1/2 inches)	1 1/2 to 2 inches
Rate	At least 100/minute	100/minute	80-100/minute
Compression to Ventilation Ratio	5:1	5:1	One-rescuer = 15:2 Two-rescuers = 5:1
Foreign-Body Airway Obstruction	Back blows/ chest thrust	Heimlich maneuver	Heimlich maneuver

Modified from: Emergency Cardiac Care Committee and Subcommittees, American Heart Association. Guidelines for cardiopulmonary resuscitation and emergency cardiac care. *JAMA* 268:2257, 1992.

26. Describe the initial management priorities for the child who is:
    a. stable
    b. in early respiratory failure
    c. in late respiratory failure
    d. in shock
    e. in cardiopulmonary failure
27. Name special conditions that predispose the infant or child to cardiopulmonary arrest.
28. State signs and symptoms of epiglottitis.
29. Name conditions that may cause respiratory failure due to trauma.
30. Name possible causes of seizures in children.

PEDIATRIC ADVANCED LIFE SUPPORT

Definition	Pediatric advanced life support refers to the assessment and support of pulmonary and circulatory function[1]
Goal	Recognize and prevent cardiopulmonary arrest

Components of Pediatric Advanced Life Support

1. Basic life support (BLS)
2. Use of adjunctive equipment and special techniques for establishing and maintaining effective ventilation and perfusion
3. Electrocardiographic (ECG) monitoring and detection of dysrhythmias
4. Establishment and maintenance of intravenous (IV) or intraosseous (IO) access
5. Treatment of patients with trauma, shock or respiratory failure
6. Therapies for emergency treatment of the patient with cardiac or respiratory arrest.

Adult vs Pediatric CPR

Major differences between cardiopulmonary resuscitation for adults and children are:

1. Sometimes dissimilar etiologies and mechanisms of arrest
    a. Most common cause of adult cardiac arrest is primarily cardiac in origin
    b. Cardiopulmonary arrest in children is usually due to profound hypoxemia and acidosis, often the result of a progressive deterioration in respiratory and circulatory function.
2. Different health professionals providing care

CARDIOPULMONARY FAILURE

Definition

Cardiopulmonary failure is a clinical condition identified by deficits in oxygenation, ventilation and perfusion, resulting in agonal respirations bradycardia, cardiopulmonary arrest.

Etiologies of Cardiopulmonary Failure[2]

Many Etiologies
|

Respiratory Distress	Early Shock
↓	↓
Respiratory Failure	Late Shock

↓

Cardiopulmonary Failure
↓
Cardiopulmonary Arrest

Multiple-Organ System Failure

Occurs when cardiac output is successfully restored but after a critical period of poor oxygen delivery, which results in substantial cellular and organ damage.

RESPIRATORY DISTRESS AND RESPIRATORY FAILURE

Definitions

1. Respiratory distress is increased work of breathing (respiratory effort)

2. Respiratory failure is a clinical condition in which there is inadequate blood oxygenation and/or ventilation to meet the metabolic demands of the body tissues

    a. Often preceded by respiratory distress in which the child's work of breathing is increased in an attempt to compensate for hypoxia
        - Increased breathing rate
        - Increased depth of breathing

    b. Primary abnormalities in respiratory failure:
        - Airway → Ventilation
        - Breathing → Oxygenation

    c. *Potential* respiratory failure is based on *clinical* observation of signs of respiratory distress.

    d. Failure of the child with potential respiratory failure to improve after initial therapy, or if signs of deterioration are observed, suggests presence of actual respiratory failure.

Precipitating Causes of
Respiratory Failure in
Infants and Children[4]

1. Infection
    a. Croup
    b. Epiglottitis
    c. Bronchiolitis
    d. Pneumonia
2. Foreign-body airway obstruction
3. Reactive airway disease
4. Smoke inhalation
5. Submersion syndrome
6. Pneumothorax and hemothorax
7. Congenital abnormalities
8. Toxin exposure
9. Neuromuscular disease
10. Congestive heart failure
11. Metabolic disease with acidosis
12. Trauma

Signs of Respiratory Distress

1. Nasal flaring
2. Inspiratory retractions
3. Increased breathing rate (tachypnea)
4. Increased depth of breathing (hyperpnea)
5. Head-bobbing
6. See-saw respirations (abdominal breathing)
7. Restlessness
8. Tachycardia
9. Grunting
10. Stridor

Signs of Respiratory Failure

1. Cyanosis
2. Diminished breath sounds
3. Decreased level of consciousness or response to pain
4. Poor skeletal muscle tone
5. Inadequate respiratory rate, effort or chest excursion
6. Tachycardia
7. Use of accessory muscles of respiration.

Table 2-1. Causes of Pediatric Cardiopulmonary Arrest

CAUSES OF PEDIATRIC CARDIOPULMONARY ARREST

Upper Respiratory	Airway Obstruction Epiglottitis Suffocation Trauma	Croup Foreign-body Strangulation
Lower Respiratory	Pneumonia Asthma Smoke inhalation Foreign-body aspiration	Bronchiolitis Near-drowning Pulmonary edema
Infection	Sepsis	Meningitis
Cardiac Disorders	Myocarditis Dysrhythmias	Pericarditis Congenital heart disease
Shock	Cardiogenic Hypovolemia with dehydration	Distributive
Neurologic	Meningitis Stroke Hypoxia	Encephalitis Head trauma
Trauma/Environment	Hypovolemia Hyperthermia	Hypothermia Near-drowning
Metabolic	Hypoglycemia Hyperkalemia	Hypocalcemia
Sudden Infant Death Syndrome (SIDS)		

Source: Barkin, R., ed., *Pediatric Emergency Medicine.* St Louis: Mosby-Year Book, 1992.

SHOCK (CIRCULATORY FAILURE)

Definition   Failure of the cardiovascular system to adequately perfuse vital organs[5]

1. "Shock may be associated with normal, low, or high cardiac output, but in all forms of shock the cardiac output is inadequate to sustain tissue perfusion and oxygen function"[6]

2. Primary abnormalities in shock:
    *   Breathing → Oxygenation
    *   Circulation → Perfusion

Table 2-2. Primary Causes of Circulatory Failure in Children;

PRIMARY CAUSES OF CIRCULATORY FAILURE IN CHILDREN

CLASSIFICATION OF SHOCK	CAUSE
Hypovolemic (loss of vascular volume)	Fluid loss • Burns • Vomiting • Diarrhea Blood loss due to trauma
Distributive (loss of peripheral vascular resistance)	Sepsis Anaphylaxis Spinal cord injury
Cardiogenic (cardiac failure)	Congenital heart disease Heart rate abnormalities Cardiomyopathy

Signs Suggestive of Early   1. Delayed capillary refill
Cardiovascular Compromise   2. Cool skin temperature
                               3. Sustained sinus tachycardia
                               4. Decreased strength of peripheral pulses
                               5. Change in level of consciousness

RESPIRATORY ASSESSMENT

EVALUATION OF THE AIRWAY

Airway → Ventilation

Rapid assessment should be performed to determine if the airway is:

1. Patent (clear)
   - If clear, no airway assistance is necessary
2. Maintainable
   - Noninvasive assistance needed
   - Head positioning
   - Suctioning
   - Use of airway adjuncts such as bag-valve-mask ventilation
3. Unmaintainable
   - Invasive intervention needed
   - Endotracheal intubation
   - Cricothyrotomy
   - Foreign body removal

EVALUATION OF BREATHING

Breathing → Oxygenation

A rapid assessment of breathing should be performed to determine:

1. Respiratory rate
2. Air Entry
   a. Stridor
   b. Prolonged expiration
   c. Breath sounds
   d. Chest expansion
3. Respiratory mechanics (work of breathing)
   a. Nasal flaring
   b. Retractions
   c. Head-bobbing
   d. See-saw respirations (abdominal breathing)
   e. Grunting
   f. Use of accessory muscles
4. Skin color and temperature

    b. May be caused by:

      1) Bronchiolitis

        a) Viral infection of the lower airway most commonly caused by the respiratory syncytial virus (RSV)

        b) Occurs primarily in infants 2-18 months of age

        c) Clinical presentation may include mild fever, runny nose, cough, wheezing

        d) May be difficult to differentiate from asthma

      2) Asthma

        a) Chronic inflammatory disease of the lower airway characterized by increased mucus production, edema and bronchospasm

        b) Uncommon before one year of age

        c) Allergic asthma may be precipitated by airborne allergens such as dust, molds, pollen and animal hair.

        d) Bronchospasm may also be triggered by anxiety, violent coughing, exercise, respiratory infections and changes in temperature

      3) Foreign body

3. Grunting

    a. Definition: partial closure of the glottis on expiration

    b. Is an attempt to build back pressure in the alveoli to maintain or increase functional residual capacity

      • Functional residual capacity is the amount of air that can be forcefully exhaled after a maximum inspiration

    c. Seen in patients with conditions resulting in collapse of the alveoli and loss of lung volume including:

      1) Pneumonia

      2) Pulmonary edema

      3) Atelectasis

      4) Adult respiratory distress syndrome

4. Breath sounds

   a. Breath sounds are normally quiet

   b. Listen along the midaxillary line in the axillae and in the mid-clavicular line under the clavicles

5. Chest rise (expansion)

   a. The chest wall should expand and contract equally with each breath

Respiratory Mechanics
(work of breathing)

- Nasal flaring
- Retractions
- Head-bobbing
- See-saw respirations (abdominal respirations)

1. Nasal flaring

   a. Widening of the nostrils on inspiration

   b. Occurs as a result of attempts to increase the size of the airway and increase the amount of available oxygen

2. Inspiratory retractions

   a. Indicate increased respiratory effort (work of breathing)

   b. Types:
      - Supraclavicular
      - Intercostal
      - Sternal
      - Substernal

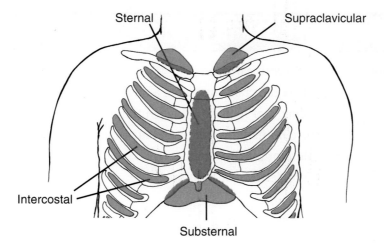

Figure 2-1. Inspiratory retractions.

3. Head bobbing
    a. Description: the head drops down with each inspiration and comes up with expansion of the chest
    b. Often an indicator of impending respiratory failure
4. See-saw (rocky) respirations (abdominal breathing)
    a. Description: inspiratory effort draws the chest in (sternal retractions) while thrusting the abdomen out
    b. Indication of severe respiratory distress

Skin Color and Temperature

1. Color reflects oxygenation and perfusion
2. Poor oxygenation results from respiratory failure and/or shock
3. Oxyhemoglobin gives arterial blood its bright red color; deoxyhemoglobin (hemoglobin that is not saturated with oxygen) gives venous blood its dark bluish color[8]
4. Cyanosis
    a. Definition: a bluish discoloration of the skin, mucous membranes and nail beds due to a lack of oxygen
    b. Seen when there are 5 or more grams per deciliter (gm/dl) of desaturated hemoglobin
    c. If the child is anemic, cyanosis may not be evident despite very low oxygen saturation
5. Cyanosis:
    a. Is best observed in the nail beds and mucous membranes of the mouth
    b. Is a very late sign of respiratory failure
    c. Peripheral cyanosis (cyanosis of the extremities) alone is more likely due to circulatory failure than pulmonary failure

MANAGEMENT OF RESPIRATORY FAILURE

Potential Respiratory Failure (Respiratory Distress)

1. Keep with caregiver
2. Allow the child to assume a position of comfort
3. Administer high flow oxygen as tolerated
4. Give nothing by mouth and maintain normal body temperature
5. Monitor pulse oximetry
6. Consider cardiac monitor

Probable Respiratory Failure

- Decreased level of consciousness
- Poor color
- Inadequate or maximal respiratory effort

1. Separate from caregiver
2. Control airway
3. Administer 100% oxygen
4. Assist ventilation if necessary
5. Give nothing by mouth
6. Monitor pulse oximetry
7. Cardiac monitor
8. Establish vascular access

CARDIOVASCULAR ASSESSMENT

Circulation → Perfusion

Rapid assessment should be performed to determine:

1. Heart rate
2. Systemic perfusion
   - peripheral pulses
   - skin perfusion
   - level of consciousness
   - urine output
3. Blood pressure

Heart Rate
(most commonly determined by palpation of the pulse)

1. Site may vary depending on the age and size of the child (brachial versus carotid or radial pulse evaluation)
2. Pulse rate variable with respirations - increases with inspiration, decreases with expiration (sinus arrhythmia)
   - Most accurate to count the pulse rate for at least 30 seconds, preferably for one full minute
3. Sinus tachycardia is a common response to many stressors such as fever, pain, anxiety, hypoxia and hypovolemia - attempt to determine the underlying cause of the tachycardia
4. Hypoxemia produces a primary response of bradycardia in the neonate; tachycardia in the older child
5. Bradycardia in the acutely ill or injured infant or child is an ominous sign of impending cardiac arrest

Table 2-4. Normal Heart Rates by Age (beats per minute)[9]

Age	Awake Rate	Sleeping Rate
Newborn to 3 months	85-205	80-160
3 months to 2 years	100-190	75-160
2 years to 10 years	60-140	60-90
>10 years	60-100	50-90

Blood Pressure

Blood pressure = cardiac output x peripheral vascular resistance

Peripheral vascular resistance = the pressure against which the heart must pump

Stroke volume = the amount of blood ejected by the left ventricle with each contraction of the heart

Cardiac output = the amount of blood pumped by the heart in one minute. Cardiac output = heart rate x stroke volume (CO = HR x SV)

Note: The proper size cuff for determining the blood pressure of a pediatric patient should be 2/3 the width of the child's upper arm.

1. An increase in either cardiac output or peripheral vascular resistance will increase blood pressure since the circulatory system is a closed system. The reverse is also true, a decrease in either cardiac output or peripheral vascular resistance will decrease blood pressure.

2. Initial compensatory mechanisms in response to shock include:
   a. Constriction of the vessels in the skin, skeletal muscle, and digestive organs in attempt to maintain perfusion of the heart, brain, and kidneys
   b. Tachycardia and increased myocardial contractility in an attempt to increase cardiac output
   c. When these compensatory mechanisms fail, hypotension occurs.

3. Hypotension
   a. Often occurs before the loss of central pulses
   b. Is preceded by a loss of perfusion of the hands and feet
   c. Is a **late and often sudden sign** of cardiovascular decompensation

Table 2-5. Normal Systolic Blood Pressure by Age[10]

Age	Systolic BP (mmHg)
0 to 1 month	60
>1 month to 1 year	70
>1 year	70 + (2 x age in years) (lower limit of normal systolic BP)

The diastolic blood pressure should be approximately 2/3 of the systolic pressure.

Reassess frequently for other signs of shock if a fall of 10 mmHg in the calculated systolic blood pressure is observed.

Peripheral Pulses

Peripheral perfusion is determined by evaluation of the presence and volume of peripheral pulses.

1. Palpation of peripheral pulses is an important part of the cardiovascular examination in determining the presence of shock.[11]
2. Pulse quality reflects adequacy of peripheral perfusion.
3. Palpation of pulses can be used to estimate:
   - Heart rate
   - Blood pressure
   - Cardiac output
   - Systemic vascular resistance
4. Palpate proximal and distal pulses simultaneously

Pulse sites

Pulse sites normally readily palpable in the healthy infant or child:
- Carotid
- Axillary
- Brachial
- Radial
- Femoral
- Dorsalis pedis
- Posterior tibial

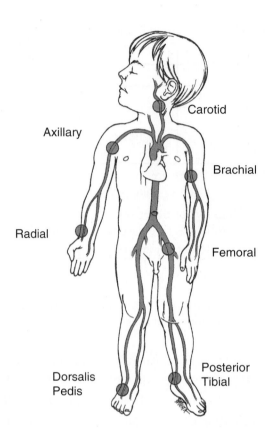

Figure 2-2. Pulse sites readily palpated in the healthy infant or child.

A difference in volume between central and peripheral pulses may be due to:

1. Hypothermia
2. An early sign of diminished stroke volume
3. Increased systemic vascular resistance

Note: Hypotension often occurs well before the loss of central pulses

Pulse Pressure
1. Definition: difference between the systolic and diastolic blood pressure
2. Indicator of stroke volume
3. Narrowed pulse pressure is an indicator of circulatory compromise

Pulse Volume
Related to pulse pressure
1. A "thready" pulse occurs as a result of narrowing pulse pressure and becomes progressively more difficult to palpate
2. Early septic shock is characterized by a wide pulse pressure, producing bounding pulses

Skin Perfusion

Evaluate:
- Extremity temperature
- Capillary refill
- Skin color

Indicators of poor skin perfusion:
- Pallor
- Mottling
- Poor capillary refill
- Peripheral cyanosis
- Decreased skin temperature

Decreased skin perfusion is an **early** sign of shock

1. Extremity temperature
   a. Cool extremities suggest inadequate cardiac output
   b. As cardiac output decreases, coolness will begin in the hands and feet and ascend toward the trunk

2. Capillary refill (consider ambient temperature)
   a. Better discriminator of shock than blood pressure in the pediatric patient
   b. Procedure: raise the extremity slightly above the level of the heart, compress the child's nail bed and release
      - If the extremity is placed in a dependent position (lower than the level of the heart), capillary refill may occur by venous refill rather than arterial flow[12]
   c. The blanched tissue should return to normal color within 2 seconds if the ambient temperature is warm
   d. Delayed capillary refill may occur as a result of low cardiac output or hypothermia
   e. If vasoconstriction of the extremities exists due to hypothermia, alternate sites for assessment of capillary refill include the gums of the mouth, forehead or sternum[13]

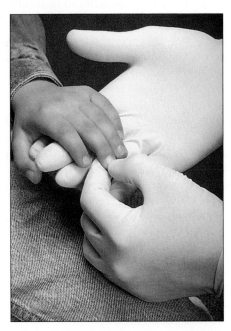

Figure 2-3. Evaluating capillary refill. (From Stoy/Center for Emergency Medicine: Mosby's EMT-Basic Textbook, St. Louis, 1996, Mosby–Year Book.)

3. Skin color

    a. Pink = normal perfusion

- Hands and feet are normally warm, dry and pink
- Newborns often have acrocyanosis (cyanotic hands and feet while the rest of the body is pink)

    b. Pale = ischemia

- Cool, pale extremities are associated with decreased cardiac output, as seen in shock and hypothermia

    c. Blue (cyanosis)

- Indicative of hypoxemia or inadequate perfusion

    d. Mottling

- Indicative of decreased cardiac output, ischemia, hypoxia

Level of Consciousness

(Central nervous system perfusion)

1. As perfusion becomes increasingly impaired, the level of responsiveness progressively deteriorates

    a. Alert - no signs or symptoms of impairment

    b. Sleepy/combative

- Sleepy while undisturbed
- Combative when procedures attempted

    c. Failure to recognize parents

- The infant should normally focus on the faces of his/her parents after 2 months of age
- Absence of parental recognition may be an early, ominous sign of decreased cortical oxygenation and/or perfusion or cerebral dysfunction

    d. Failure to respond to pain

    e. Fluctuating level of consciousness

2. The acronym AVPU is used to objectively describe the level of consciousness:

A = **A**wake

V = response to **V**erbal (voice) stimuli

P = response to **P**ainful stimuli

U = **U**nresponsive

3. Deep tendon reflexes may be depressed

4. Pupils may be small but reactive

5. Cheyne-Stokes breathing pattern may be apparent

    a. Characterized by alternating periods of apnea and deep, fast breathing

    b. Breathing slowly becomes shallower, climaxing in a 10 to 20 second period without breathing before the cycle is repeated. Each cycle may last from 45 seconds to 3 minutes.[14]

Urine Output
(Kidney Perfusion)

1. Urine output reflects glomerular filtration rate → renal blood flow → kidney perfusion

2. Normal = 1-2 ml/kg/hr

3. Urine output of less than 1 ml/kg/hr, in the absence of renal disease, is a sign of poor perfusion

4. Placement of an indwelling urinary catheter assists in determining accurate urine output and kidney perfusion

5. Rate of urinary flow is a good indicator in evaluating the success of volume expansion

CLASSIFICATIONS OF SHOCK

Hypovolemic Shock

1. Most common cause of shock in children

2. Normal blood volume[15]

    a. Premature neonate average = 90-105 ml/kg

    b. Term newborn average = 85 ml/kg

    c. Children over 1 month to 11 months of age average = 75 ml/kg

    d. Beyond one year of age average = 65 to 75 ml/kg in children

    e. Adult average = 55 to 57 ml/kg

3. A loss of 10-15% of circulating blood volume, in a healthy child, is usually well tolerated and easily compensated.

4. Signs of early, compensated shock:

    a. Increased heart rate

    b. Cutaneous vasoconstriction

      • Skin mottling

      • Delayed capillary refill

      • Cool extremities

    c. Diminished pulse pressure

    d. Blood pressure is frequently normal

    e. Normal or minimally impaired neurologic status

3. An acute loss of 25% or more of the circulating blood volume (eg. moderate hemorrhage) usually produces signs and symptoms of decompensated shock characterized by:

  a. Hypotension

    • Hypotension occurs when compensatory mechanisms have been exhausted

  b. Significant tachycardia

  c. Delayed capillary refill

  d. Altered mental status - irritability, lethargy

  e. Decreased urine output

  f. Weak central pulses

  g. Cool extremities, mottling or pallor

Distributive Shock

1. Sepsis

  a. Definition: evidence of an infection and a systemic response[16]

  b. Clinical signs

    • Evidence of infection

    • Tachycardia

    • Tachypnea

    • Fever or hypothermia

    • Possible peripheral vasodilation

2. Sepsis (or septic) syndrome

  a. Definition: evidence of sepsis with evidence of altered organ perfusion[17]

  b. Clinical signs

    • Signs of sepsis plus signs of altered organ perfusion

    • Pulmonary failure

      • Increased work of breathing, respiratory acidosis, or intrapulmonary shunting

      • GI/hepatic dysfunction

        • GI ulceration or bleeding, paralytic ileus, elevation in liver enzymes, coagulopathy

      • Oliguria or renal failure

3. Septic shock

  a. Definition: sepsis syndrome with hypotension[18]

  b. Clinical signs

    • Signs of sepsis syndrome with hypotension

4. Anaphylaxis
   a. Definition: a severe allergic response to a foreign substance with which the patient has had prior contact
   b. Clinical signs
      • Stridor, wheezing, hoarseness, intercostal and suprasternal retractions
      • Tachycardia, hypotension, dysrhythmias
      • Vomiting, diarrhea
      • Angioedema
      • Urticaria

Cardiogenic Shock

1. Cardiogenic shock may be seen:[19]
   a. After cardiovascular surgery
   b. With inflammatory cardiac diseases
      • Cardiomyopathy
      • Myocarditis
   c. With severe congenital heart disease
   d. As a result of drug toxicity, severe electrolyte or acid-base imbalances

2. Cardiogenic shock occurs as a result of the inability of the cardiovascular system to meet the metabolic needs of body tissues. Although cardiogenic shock may be due to an underlying cardiac disorder, it may also occur as a complication of shock of any cause.

3. Signs and symptoms are usually the result of low cardiac output:
   a. Delayed capillary refill
   b. Cool extremities (cooling will begin in the periphery and ascend toward the trunk)
   c. Mottling of the skin
   d. Diminished peripheral pulses

Stages of Shock

1. Early (compensated) shock
   a. Increase in heart rate and myocardial contractility
   b. Increase in peripheral vascular resistance
   c. Pulse pressure narrows

2. Late (uncompensated) shock
   a. Compensatory mechanisms fail
   b. Blood pressure falls, compromising blood flow to vital organs

　　　　　　　　　　　3.　Irreversible shock

　　　　　　　　　　　　　a.　Cellular death begins, ultimately resulting in multiple-organ system failure

　　　　　　　　　　　　　b.　Even if the patient is resuscitated during this stage, long-term survival is unlikely due to end-organ failure (kidneys, lungs, liver, heart) days later.

Management of Shock　　　1.　Rapidly establish vascular access

　　　　　　　　　　　　　a.　In hemorrhagic shock, establish at least two lines

　　　　　　　　　　　　　b.　The cannula used should be of short length and large-gauge

　　　　　　　　　　　2.　Volume expansion - 20 ml/kg crystalloid solution initial bolus (in less than 20 minutes) in hypovolemic shock

　　　　　　　　　　　3.　Vasoactive infusions

　　　　　　　　　　　4.　Administer high concentration oxygen

　　　　　　　　　　　5.　Place on a cardiorespiratory monitor

　　　　　　　　　　　6.　Place on pulse oximeter

　　　　　　　　　　　7.　Maintain normothermia

RAPID CARDIOPULMONARY ASSESSMENT

Description and Purpose
- 30-second survey
- Designed to evaluate pulmonary and cardiovascular function and their effects on end-organ perfusion and function[20]

Components
1. Physical examination
2. Evaluation of physiologic status
3. Initial management priorities

Conditions Requiring Rapid Cardiopulmonary Assessment[21]
- Respiratory rate greater than 60
- Heart rate greater than 180 or less than 80 (5 years or less)
- Heart rate greater than 160 or less than 60 (over 5 years)
- Increased work of breathing (retractions, nasal flaring, grunting)
- Trauma
- Burns totaling > 10% of body surface area
- Cyanosis or a decrease in oxyhemoglobin saturation
- Altered level of consciousness (unusual irritability, lethargy, or failure)
- Seizures
- Fever with petechiae (small hemorrhages of the skin)

PHYSICAL EXAMINATION

Purpose   Ascertain the presence of respiratory failure or shock

Phases

1. Initial evaluation of the ABCs (primary assessment)
   a. Inspection of the airway
   b. Evaluation of breathing
   c. Palpation of peripheral pulses
2. Secondary evaluation
   a. Assessment of heart rate, respiratory rate and blood pressure
   b. Determination of level of consciousness
   c. Auscultation of breath sounds

EVALUATION OF PHYSIOLOGIC STATUS

Purpose   To determine the severity of change in the patient's physiologic condition

Patient Condition

1. Stable
2. Respiratory failure
   - Potential
   - Probable
3. Shock
   - Compensated
   - Decompensated
4. Cardiopulmonary failure
   - Leads to agonal respirations, bradycardia, cardiopulmonary arrest

INITIAL MANAGEMENT PRIORITIES

Purpose   To determine priorities in patient management based on the physical examination findings and physiologic status evaluation

Patient Categories

1. Stable
2. Questionable respiratory failure or shock
3. Definite respiratory failure or shock
4. Cardiopulmonary failure

Management of the
Stable Patient

1. Begin further work-up
   - Laboratory studies
   - Arterial blood gases
   - Chest roentgenogram
2. Provide specific therapy as indicated
3. Reassess frequently

Management of Potential Respiratory Failure	1. Keep with caregiver
	2. Position of comfort
	3. Oxygen as tolerated
	4. Give nothing by mouth
	5. Monitor pulse oximetry
	6. Consider cardiac monitor

Management of Potential Respiratory Failure

1. Keep with caregiver
2. Position of comfort
3. Oxygen as tolerated
4. Give nothing by mouth
5. Monitor pulse oximetry
6. Consider cardiac monitor

Management of Probable Respiratory Failure

1. Separate from caregiver
2. Control the airway
3. Administer 100% oxygen
4. Assist ventilation
5. Give nothing by mouth
6. Monitor pulse oximetry
7. Cardiac monitor
8. Establish vascular access

Management of Shock

1. Administer 100% oxygen and ensure adequate airway and ventilation
2. Establish vascular access
3. Provide volume expansion
4. Monitor oxygenation, heart rate, and urine output
5. Consider vasoactive infusions

Management of Cardiopulmonary Failure

1. Oxygenate, ventilate, and monitor
2. Reassess for respiratory failure and shock
   - Patient's response to drug therapy may help determine if the underlying cause of cardiopulmonary failure is respiratory failure or shock
3. Establish vascular access

SPECIAL CONDITIONS PREDISPOSING TO CARDIOPULMONARY ARREST

Positive-Pressure Ventilation

Hypoxemia may result in cardiopulmonary arrest despite intubation of the trachea and positive-pressure ventilation if:

- The endotracheal tube is obstructed
- The endotracheal tube is displaced into the esophagus or mainstem bronchus
- A tension pneumothorax is present
- The mechanical ventilation device fails

Epiglottitis

1. Usually presents before the age of 5 years
2. Signs and symptoms:
   - High fever
   - Sore throat
   - Drooling
   - Dyspnea
   - Muffled voice
   - Inspiratory stridor
   - Tripod position (leaning forward while sitting and holding the head in a sniffing position)
3. Respiratory arrest may occur as a result of:
   - Total airway obstruction
   - Combination of partial airway obstruction and fatigue

Management:

1. Position of comfort
2. Avoid upsetting the child, allow the caregiver to hold the child while supplemental oxygen is administered
3. Do not attempt to visualize the airway or perform any invasive treatments
   - The child should be taken directly to the operating room for controlled intubation if epiglottitis is strongly suspected
4. Perform bag-mask ventilation with 100% oxygen if respiratory arrest occurs prior to any intubation attempts, tracheotomy or needle cricothyrotomy

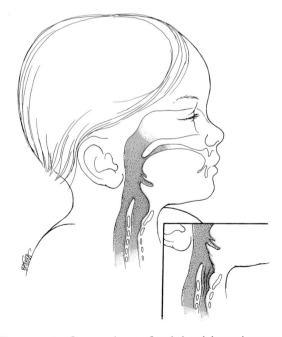

Figure 2-4. Comparison of epiglottitis and croup.

Table 2-6. Comparison of Croup and Epiglottitis.

COMPARISON OF CROUP AND EPIGLOTTITIS

	CROUP	EPIGLOTTITIS
Age	3 months to 3 years	3 to 7 years
Location	Subglottic	Supraglottic
Onset	Gradual	Sudden
Organism	Viral	Bacterial
Fever	100-101°F	102-104°F
Signs and Symptoms	Barking cough	Drooling
	Retractions	Retractions
	Hoarse voice	Muffled voice
	Harsh cough	Usually no cough
	Loud stridor	Prefers to sit up and learn forward to breathe (tripod position)

Tracheostomy

1. An infant experiencing obstruction of his/her tracheostomy tube due to a mucous plug is at high risk for respiratory arrest.

2. An arrest in a patient with a tracheostomy should be presumed to be due to tracheal obstruction until proven otherwise.

3. If suctioning attempts fail to relieve the obstruction, immediately remove the tracheostomy tube.

   • The infant often has enough reserve to breathe spontaneously before the stoma is suctioned and a new tube is inserted[22]

   • The stoma can be manually occluded and ventilation performed with a bag-mask device before orotracheal intubation is attempted

Burns

1. Children who have suffered major burns should be reevaluated frequently for respiratory failure and shock.

2. The decision to perform endotracheal intubation should be made early in the management of the child who has suffered severe burns of the head and neck or in cases of inhalation injury since swelling occurs rapidly and may cause airway occlusion.

3. Carbon monoxide poisoning should be treated with maximum supplemental oxygen.

Trauma

Respiratory failure due to trauma may occur as a result of:

- Flail chest
- Pneumothorax
- Pulmonary contusion
- Upper airway obstruction
- Central nervous system depression

Hemorrhagic shock is most often due to injury to the liver or spleen. Other sites of major blood loss include:

- Hemothorax
- Scalp lacerations
- Intracranial hemorrhage (newborn or infant)
- Fractured femur with vascular laceration

Suspected fractures of the cervical spine should be treated with cervical spine immobilization until evidence of fracture has been ruled out.

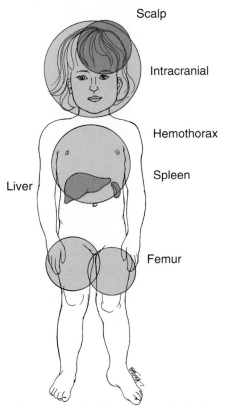

Figure 2-5. Sites of major blood loss due to trauma.

Gastroenteritis

1. The presence of a gastrointestinal infection may result in shock due to hypovolemia.
2. Signs of dehydration precede shock.
3. Rapid volume expansion is necessary to prevent cardiovascular collapse.

Table 2-7. Signs and Symptoms of Dehydration.

DEHYDRATION SEVERITY

Assessment	Mild	Moderate	Severe
Vital Signs			
Heart rate	Normal	Increased	Tachycardia > 130/min
Respiratory rate	Normal	Increased	Tachypnea
Blood pressure	Normal	Normal	Hypotensive, systolic < 80
Capillary refill	Normal	2-3 seconds	> 3 seconds
Mental Status	Alert	Irritable	Lethargic
Skin			
Color	Pale	Ashen	Mottled
Turgor	Normal	Poor	Tenting
Temperature	Warm	Cool	Cool, clammy
Texture	Normal	Dry	Doughy
Fontanelle	Flat	Depressed	Sunken
Mucous Membranes	Dry	Very dry	Parched
	± tears	No tears	
Eyes	Normal	Darkened	Sunken
	Sunken	Soft	
Thirst	Increased	Intense	Intense if conscious
Urine Output	Normal	Decreased	Minimal
	Concentrated	Very concentrated	

Source: Eichelberger M: *Pediatric Emergencies: A Manual for Prehospital Care Providers*, Englewood Cliffs, Prentice-Hall, 1992.

Seizures

Causes of seizures in children

1. Toxic/metabolic causes
   - Hypoxia
   - Dehydration
   - Hypoglycemia
   - Electrolyte imbalance
   - Toxic ingestion or exposure
2. Tumors
3. Trauma
   - Subarachnoid hemorrhage
   - Subdural or epidural hematoma
4. Infection
   - Meningitis
   - Encephalitis
5. Other
   - Fever
   - Epilepsy
   - Failure to take antiseizure medication

Seizures may result in:

1. Respiratory depression
2. Upper airway obstruction due to:
   - Secretions
   - Prolapse of soft tissues into the hypopharynx

Critically Ill Child

Infants and children in an intensive care unit, operating room, emergency department or in transit between hospitals are at high risk for cardiopulmonary arrest[23] which may occur as a result of:

- the natural history of a life-threatening disease
- a complication of therapy
- premature withdrawal of support, including mechanical ventilation, supplemental oxygen or vasoactive drugs
- the accidental withdrawal of support.

Cardiac arrest may recur in the recently resuscitated child due to:

- catecholamines administered during resuscitation that have been metabolized and not replaced by a continuous infusion
- recurrence of the inciting event
- hypoxic-ischemic myocardial, pulmonary or cerebral damage has occurred

Coma

1. Intubation is necessary to protect the airway and treat hypoventilation in the comatose infant or child.

    •   Essential that intubation be performed by skilled personnel

2. Posturing observed after head trauma should be considered a sign of increased intracranial pressure

    •   Decorticate posturing - the legs are extended and the arms flexed

    •   Decerebrate posturing - the extremities are extended and the arms rotated inward

3. Cushing's triad is a LATE sign of increased intracranial pressure

    •   Irregular respiration or apnea

    •   Bradycardia

    •   Hypertension

Note: The absence of Cushing's triad does not rule out the presence of increased intracranial pressure.

Decorticate

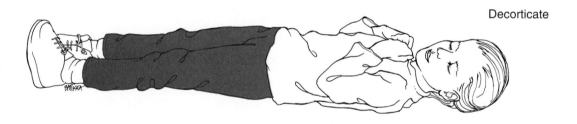

Decerebrate

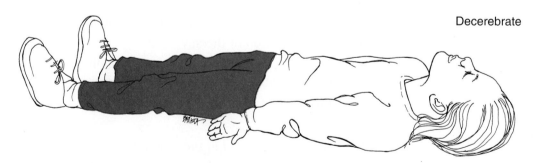

Figure 2-6. Decorticate and decerebrate posturing.

REFERENCES

1. Emergency Cardiac Care Committee and Subcommittees, American Heart Association. Guidelines for cardiopulmonary resuscitation and emergency cardiac care. *JAMA* 268:2262, 1992.

2. Quan L, Seidel JS (ed.), *Instructor's Manual for Pediatric Advanced Life Support.* Dallas: American Heart Association, 1995, p. 4-1.

3. Quan L, Seidel JS (ed.), *Instructor's Manual for Pediatric Advanced Life Support.* Dallas: American Heart Association, 1995, p. 4-7.

4. Barkin, R., (ed.), *Pediatric Emergency Medicine.* St. Louis: Mosby-Year Book, 1992.

5. Crone RK. Acute circulatory failure in children. *Pediatr Clin North Am* 27:525, 1980.

6. Barkin, R., (ed.), *Pediatric Emergency Medicine.* St. Louis: Mosby-Year Book, 1992.

7. Hazinski, MF. *Children are different. Nursing Care of the Critically Ill Child.* 2nd ed. St. Louis: Mosby-Year Book, 1992.

8. Carroll PL. Cyanosis, the sign you can't count on, *Nursing88* 18(3):50, 1988.

9. Gillette PC, Garson A, Jr, Porter CJ, McNamara DG. Dysrhythmias. In Adams FH, Emmanouilides GC, Riemenschneider TA (ed.), *Moss' Heart Disease in Infants, Children, and Adolescents,* ed 4, Baltimore: Williams & Wilkins, 1989, p. 725-741.

10. Quan L, Seidel JS (ed.), *Instructor's Manual for Pediatric Advanced Life Support.* Dallas: American Heart Association, 1995, p. 4-6.

11. Quan L, Seidel JS (ed.), *Instructor's Manual for Pediatric Advanced Life Support.* Dallas: American Heart Association, 1995, p. 4-5.

12. Quan L, Seidel JS (ed.), *Instructor's Manual for Pediatric Advanced Life Support.* Dallas: American Heart Association, 1995, p. 4-6.

13. Eichelberger M. *Pediatric Emergencies: A Manual for Prehospital Care Providers,* Englewood Cliffs, Prentice-Hall, 1992.

14. Yvorra, J (ed.), *Mosby's Emergency Dictionary.* St. Louis: C. V. Mosby Company, 1989.

15. Fuhrman, B. *Pediatric Critical Care.* St. Louis: Mosby-Year Book, 1992.

19. Of the following, which finding would most accurately reflect brain hypoperfusion?

a. tachycardia
b. hypotension
c. pupillary dilation
d. altered level of consciousness

20. On the basis of physical examination findings and physiologic status evaluation, the pediatric patient is categorized as:

1. _____

2. _____

3. _____

4. _____

14		Respiratory
		occur as a r
		pneumotho
		upper airwa
		nervous sys
15	C	The formul:
		lower limit
		pressure in
		years is 70
		Thus, 70 +
16	B	This child's
		onset of fe
		tripod posi
		epiglottitis
17	C	During CPF
		should be
		approxima
		depth of tl
		1 1/2 inche
18	A	Causes of
		include co
		tumor or
		infections
		body aspir
		olitis may
		airway.
19	D	An altered
		early indic
		Pupillary
		signs are
		significan
20		On the ba
		assessmer
		1. Stable
		2. In resp
		• Pote
		• Prob
		3. In sho
		• Con
		• Dec
		4. In card

QUIZ ANSWERS – RESPIRATORY FAILURE, SHOCK, AND BASIC LIFE SUPPORT

QUESTION	ANSWER	RATIONALE	STUDY GUIDE PAGE REFERENCE	PALS PAGE REFERENCE
1	A	Hypoxemia produces a primary response of bradycardia in the neonate; tachycardia in the older child.	53	2-5
2		The acronym AVPU is used to objectively classify level of consciousness: A = Awake V = responds to Verbal stimuli P = responds to Painful stimuli U = Unresponsive	58	2-6
3	C	Normal urine output = 1-2 ml/kg/hr This child weighs 33 pounds (15 kg), therefore, normal urine output for this child for one hour would be 15-30 ml, 60-120 ml for a four hour period. Urine output of less than 1 ml/kg/hr, in the absence of renal disease, is a sign of poor perfusion.	59	2-6
4	B	Minute volume is the amount of air inhaled and exhaled in one minute. It is the product of tidal volume and respiratory rate. (Minute volume = tidal volume x respiratory rate).	48	2-2
5	B	In compensated shock the blood pressure is normal. Decompensated shock is characterized by hypotension and, often, low cardiac output (suggests a loss of at least 20% of circulating blood volume).	61	2-2
6	D	90 + (2 x age in years) is the formula used to approximate the median systolic blood pressure in children over the age of 1 year.	55	2-5

7	C	The re openi suspe and s
8	A	"Quie descri distres maint diseas diarrh renal metab
9		Indica includ refill, skin t
10	D	Prolor bronch bronch usuall Strido obstru patien collap volum pneum respira
11	C	Hemo injury of maj scalp l rhage femur
12		Septic types by an norma
13	A	Ventila maneu child.

Mechanism of Breathing

1. Respiratory centers are located in the medulla and pons. The respiratory muscles receive impulses from the medulla.
   a. The phrenic nerve stimulates the diaphragm.
   b. Intercostal nerves stimulate the external intercostal muscles.
2. Primary muscles of respiration
   a. Diaphragm
      1) Dome-shaped muscle below the lungs
      2) Flattens and moves downward when it contracts
      3) Tidal volume in the pediatric patient is more dependent on the function and movement of the diaphragm
         - The muscles of the chest wall are not well-developed in the child
         - Effective respiration may be jeopardized when diaphragmatic movement is compromised since the chest wall cannot compensate
   b. External intercostal muscles
      1) Pull the ribs upward and outward
      2) Chest cavity is expanded from front to back and side-to-side during inspiration
   c. Internal intercostal muscles
      1) Located between the ribs
      2) Pull the ribs downward and inward

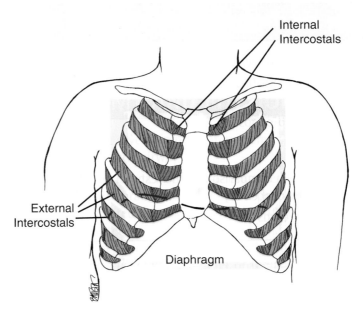

Figure 3-1. The primary muscles of respiration.

3. The lungs are supported and protected by the ribs.

   a. The chest wall of the infant and young child is pliable as it is composed of more cartilage than bone.

   b. As a result of the flexibility of the ribs, children are more resistant to rib fractures than adults, though the force of the injury is readily transmitted to the delicate tissues of the lung which may result in pulmonary contusion or hemopneumothorax.

   c. Due to their pliability, the ribs may fail to support the lung leading to paradoxical movement (sternal and intercostal retractions) during active inspiration, rather than lung expansion.

Metabolic Rate   Oxygen demands of the pediatric patient are 2-3 times that of an adult.

- 6-8 ml/kg/min in a child
- 3-4 ml/kg/min in the adult

OXYGEN DELIVERY SYSTEMS

General Principles

1. Supplemental humidified oxygen should be supplied in the highest concentration available to the infant or child with acute respiratory distress.

   a. Humidified oxygen helps prevent drying of the mucous membranes and loosens secretions.

   b. Cool mist systems may produce hypothermia in the small child, therefore, heated humidification systems are preferred.

2. Monitoring of patients with chronic respiratory insufficiency (advanced cystic fibrosis, bronchopulmonary dysplasia) is essential since administration of high flow oxygen to these patients may abolish their respiratory drive.

Indications for Oxygen Administration

1. All cases of cardiopulmonary arrest

2. Suspected hypoxemia of any cause

3. Any condition of respiratory difficulty that may lead to cardiac arrest

NASAL CANNULA (NASAL PRONGS)

Description and Function

1. Plastic tubing with two ports designed to deliver supplemental oxygen through the nares
2. Low-flow oxygen delivery system
3. Can deliver oxygen concentrations of approximately 25-45% at 1-6 liters/minute
   - The actual inspired oxygen concentration is dependent on a number of factors including oxygen flow rate, tidal volume and inspiratory flow rate

Advantages

1. Easy to use
2. Lightweight
3. Disposable
4. Useful for the child with moderate oxygen needs

Disadvantages

1. Oxygen flow rates of greater than 4 liters/minute are irritating to the nose and throat
2. Can deliver only a relatively low concentration of oxygen
3. Adequate humidification cannot be provided by means of this device
4. Can only be used in the spontaneously breathing patient

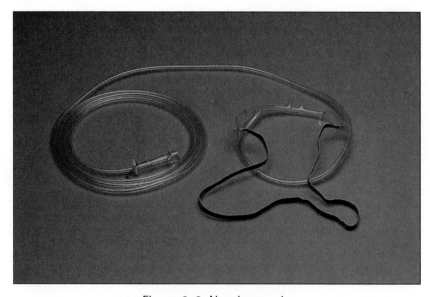

Figure 3-2. Nasal cannula.

NASAL CATHETER

Description and Function | Flexible oxygen catheter with multiple holes in the distal tip which is placed into one naris and advanced posteriorly into the pharynx behind the uvula.

Advantages | None over the nasal cannula

Disadvantages | Use of this device is discouraged.

1. May cause hemorrhage as a result of trauma to enlarged adenoids.

2. May produce gastric distention or rupture if inadvertently placed in the esophagus.

OXYGEN HOOD

Description and Function

1. Clear plastic dome that encircles the child's head.

2. Permits control of oxygen concentration, temperature and humidity.

3. Can deliver up to 100% oxygen with oxygen flow rates of 10-15 liters/minute.

4. Oxygen flow rate must be at least 6 liters/minute to avoid the accumulation of exhaled air in the hood.

Advantages

1. Permits access to the chest, trunk and extremities for continued care.

2. Well-tolerated by infants.

Disadvantages

1. Very noisy for the patient

2. Generally not large enough to be used with children over the age of 1 year.

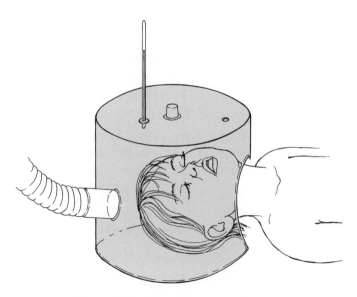

Figure 3-3. The oxygen hood.

OXYGEN TENT

Description and Function	1. Clear plastic shell that surrounds the entire child
	2. Can deliver an oxygen concentration of 21-50%
Advantages	Provides a method of increased oxygen delivery
Disadvantages	1. Limited accessibility to the child
	2. Reduction in oxygen concentration due to outside air entering the tent when accessing the child
	3. Very noisy for the patient
	4. Difficult to observe the child if a cool mist is used

SIMPLE FACE MASK (STANDARD MASK)

Description and Function	1. Plastic device with several small holes on each side that allows for inhalation and exhalation of air. There is also a port for delivery of supplemental oxygen on the lower portion of the mask.
	a. Air holes on the sides of the mask allow passage of inspired **and** expired air
	b. Supplemental oxygen is directed into the mask
	c. Concentration of inspired oxygen is less than that with a nonrebreather mask because the supplemental oxygen mixes with room air.
	2. The oxygen flow rate must be higher than 6 liters/minute to avoid the accumulation of exhaled air in the mask reservoir that might be rebreathed.
	3. Recommended flow rate is 6-10 liters/minute. At this flow rate, the device provides approximately 35-60% oxygen.
Advantages	Higher oxygen concentration delivered than by nasal cannula
Disadvantages	1. Usually not well tolerated by infants
	2. Variability in actual inspired oxygen concentration (this is because the amount of air that mixes with supplemental oxygen is dependent upon the patient's inspiratory flow rate)
	3. Because of the variability in delivered FiO_2 with this mask, a nonrebreather mask may be preferable when high concentrations of oxygen are required
	4. Not tolerated well in the severely dyspneic child (feeling of suffocation)
	5. Can only be used with spontaneously breathing patients

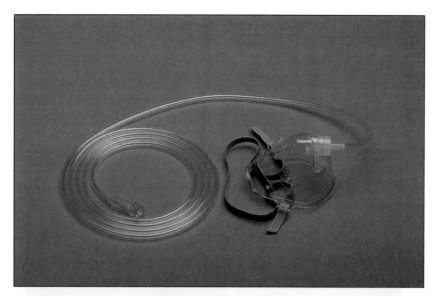

Figure 3-4. Simple face mask.

PARTIAL REBREATHING MASK

Description and Function	Can deliver an FiO_2 of 50-60% at 10-12 liters/minute oxygen flow with a good face-mask seal.

1. Consists of a simple face mask with a reservoir bag
2. The patient inhales oxygen from the reservoir bag and, potentially, room air from the exhalation ports on the mask

Advantages	Higher oxygen concentrations delivered than with the nasal cannula or simple face mask
Disadvantages	Can only be used with spontaneously breathing patients
Special Considerations	

1. The reservoir bag must remain completely inflated when using this device so sufficient supplemental oxygen is available for each breath
2. Must use oxygen flow rates of 10-12 liters/minute

NONREBREATHING MASK

Description and Function	Can deliver an FiO_2 of up to 95% at 10-12 liters/minute oxygen flow with a good face-mask seal

1. A one-way valve is present on one side of the nonrebreather mask that allows exhaled air to escape but prevents room air from being inspired
2. Supplemental oxygen is directed into the reservoir bag of the nonrebreather device
3. The patient inhales 100% oxygen from the reservoir bag

Advantages	Higher oxygen concentration delivered than with the nasal cannula or simple face mask

Technique - Two Rescuers　　　One person holds the mask to the face with two hands while maintaining an open airway and a second rescuer compresses the ventilation bag.

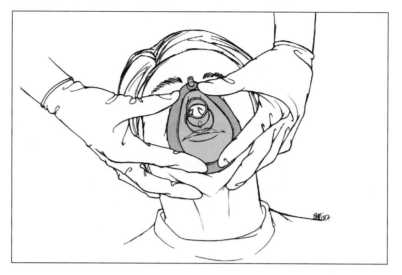

Figure 3-12. Ventilating with a bag-valve device - two-rescuer technique.
A second rescuer compresses the ventilation bag.

Special Considerations

1. While ventilating, monitor the patient for improvement in heart rate, color, pulses, perfusion, and blood pressure

2. If an air leak is present with ventilation due to an improper seal, reposition the mask. If the leak persists:

   a. Ask for assistance with the airway

   b. Consider using another mask

   c. Use the two-hand technique

3. Gastric distention can be minimized by providing adequate inspiratory time (1-1$\frac{1}{2}$ seconds per breath) with each compression of the bag.

4. Cricoid pressure may be used in the unconscious patient to minimize gastric distention and aspiration.

5. The bag-valve device should only be used by trained operators.

Positive End-Expiratory Pressure (PEEP)

Positive end-expiratory pressure is used to deliver positive pressure during expiration, preventing the collapse of the alveoli during expiration.

PEEP therapy is used to:[10]

1. Increase functional residual capacity

2. Reexpand collapsed and partially collapsed alveoli

3. Decrease right-to-left intrapulmonary shunting of blood

4. Improve ventilation/perfusion imbalances

5. Improve oxygenation so that toxic concentrations of oxygen are no longer required.

PEEP is used in the management of disease processes that result in alveolar collapse, impairing oxygenation as in:

1. Aspiration
2. Pneumonia
3. Atelectasis
4. Pulmonary edema
5. Adult respiratory distress syndrome

ANESTHESIA VENTILATION SYSTEMS

Description and Function
1. Inflates only when air or oxygen from a compressed gas source is forced into it.
2. Consists of an anesthesia bag, exhaust valve, 15/22 mm adaptor for connection to a mask or tracheal tube, a fresh gas inlet and a piece of plastic tubing. Some models also have a site for attachment of a pressure-gauge.

Advantages
1. Provides a continuous flow of oxygen for the spontaneously breathing patient.
2. Sense of lung compliance conveyed to the operator
3. More reliable control of oxygen concentration delivered

   Since the oxygen entering the bag does not mix with room air (as in the self-inflating bag), the oxygen concentration entering the bag is the same concentration delivered to the patient
4. Can deliver CPAP (continuous positive airway pressure) or PEEP (positive end-expiratory pressure)

Disadvantages
1. Requires continuous air-oxygen flow to operate
2. Should be used only by individuals trained and experienced in the use of the device

Complications
Barotrauma

Tension pneumothorax

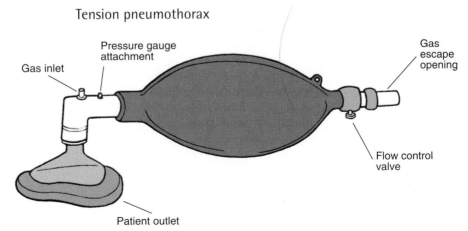

Figure 3-13. Anesthesia bag.

OXYGEN-POWERED BREATHING DEVICES

Description

1. Consists of a high-pressure tubing connecting the oxygen supply and a valve that is activated by a lever or push button; when the valve is open, oxygen flows into the patient.
2. Allows positive-pressure ventilation with 100% oxygen.

Contraindications

Not recommended for use in the pediatric patient because tidal volume is difficult to control and excessive airway pressures may develop, resulting in gastric distention or tension pneumothorax.

ENDOTRACHEAL INTUBATION

Advantages

1. Prevents gastric distention and reduces the risk of aspiration by isolating the larynx and trachea from the pharynx, ensuring adequate ventilation and delivery of oxygen.
2. Permits suctioning of airway secretions, blood, mucus or meconium.
3. Provides a route for administration of some medications when intravenous access cannot be obtained.
   - LEAN or LANE = Lidocaine, Atropine, Naloxone, Epinephrine
4. Permits control of inspiratory time and peak inspiratory pressures
5. Permits delivery of positive end-expiratory pressure (PEEP)

Indications[11]

1. Inadequate central nervous system control of ventilation
2. Functional or anatomic airway obstruction
3. Excessive work of breathing leading to fatigue and respiratory insufficiency.
4. Need for high peak inspiratory pressure or positive end-expiratory pressure to maintain effective alveolar gas exchange
5. Need for mechanical ventilatory support
6. Potential occurence of any of the above if patient transport is needed.

Endotracheal Tube

1. Should be sterile and disposable
2. Should be of uniform internal diameter
3. Should possess a standard 15 mm adaptor at the proximal end for attachment to a ventilating device

4. Should have cm markings for use as reference points
   - Aids in placement of the endotracheal tube
   - Assists in detecting accidental movement of the tube
5. Distal end may include a Murphy eye (hole in the side wall of the tube)
   - Helps prevent complete tube occlusion if the end opening of the endotracheal tube should become blocked
6. Cuffed endotracheal tubes can be used in children greater than 8 years of age
   - A high-volume, low-pressure cuff should be used to prevent damage to the tissue mucosa
7. In children under the age of 8 years, an uncuffed endotracheal tube should be used
   - The narrowing at the level of the cricoid cartilage serves as a natural cuff for the endotracheal tube
8. Estimation of endotracheal tube size is best based on patient size, rather than age
   - The internal diameter of the endotracheal tube is approximately equal to the diameter of the child's little finger
   - The Broselow Resuscitation Tape is useful in identifying the proper endotracheal tube size for a child of any age
   - For children older than 1 year of age, the following formulas may be used:

$$\text{Tube size (mm I.D.)} = \frac{\text{age (years)} + 4}{4} \quad \text{or} \quad \frac{16 + \text{patient's age in years}}{4}$$

   - For children less than 1 year of age, no single formula is completely reliable. For most premature infants, a 2.5-3.0 mm tube may be used; 3.5 mm for older infants.

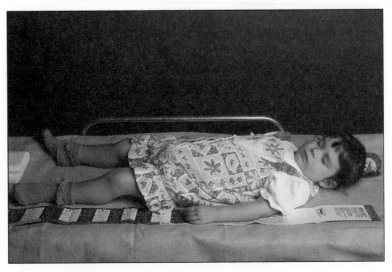

Figure 3-14. The Broselow resuscitation tape.

Laryngoscope Blades

1. May be straight or curved

   a. The straight blade directly lifts the epiglottis.

      • The straight blade is preferred in infants and children up to the age of 7-8 years because the blade provides greater movement of the large tongue into the floor of the mouth and visualization of the glottic opening.

   b. The tip of the curved blade is inserted into the vallecula. The soft tissue is then lifted and the glottic opening (the space between the vocal cords) is visualized.

      • Vallecula means "little valley" and is the space between the base of the tongue and the epiglottis.

      • The curved blade is preferred in the older child because the broader base and flange of the blade aid displacement of the tongue.

      • The curved blade must be chosen more carefully to fit the size of the tongue.

2. Blade size can be determined by:

   • holding the blade next to the patient's face. The proper blade size will extend from the patient's lips to the Adam's apple

   • Broselow tape®

   • Better to choose a blade that is too long than too short

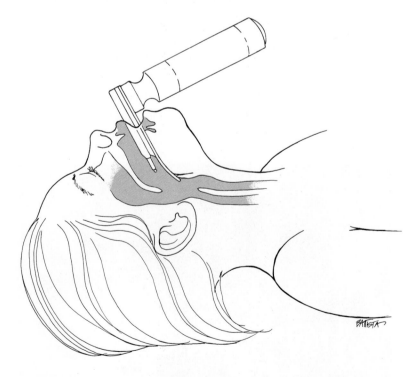

Figure 3-15. The straight blade directly lifts the epiglottis.

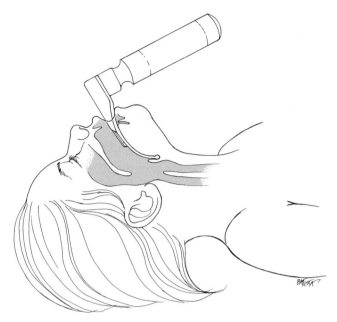

Figure 3-16. The tip of the curved blade is inserted into the vallecula.

Equipment

1. Body substance isolation precautions (Gloves, mask, protective eye wear)

2. Oxygen source

3. Tonsil-tip suction and endotracheal suction catheter available

4. Endotracheal tube of appropriate size plus $1/2$ size larger and $1/2$ size smaller

5. Laryngoscope handle and blade with a functioning "white, bright light"

6. Bag-valve device with ventilation mask of appropriate size

7. Stylet

   - The stylet is a metal wire (may be plastic-coated) inserted inside the endotracheal tube that provides rigidity to the endotracheal tube and allows the tube to be shaped to any desired configuration, facilitating placement of the endotracheal tube through the vocal cords

   - Some advocate lubrication of the stylet with a water-soluble lubricant prior to placement in the endotracheal tube to aid removal once the tube has been placed, avoiding accidental extubation

8. Materials for securing the endotracheal tube

9. Pulse oximeter

   - A pulse oximeter should be used whenever possible during intubation

Procedure

1. Assure the child is being adequately ventilated prior to the intubation attempt

2. If a cuffed endotracheal tube is used, check the tube cuff for leaks

3. If a stylet is used, assure the tip of the stylet is recessed 1-2 cm from the end of the endotracheal tube to avoid trauma to the anatomical structures

4. Connect the laryngoscope blade and handle

5. Attain proper head position

    a. Three axes must be aligned to achieve direct visualization of the larynx (mouth, pharynx and trachea).

    b. This is accomplished when the head is placed in a "sniffing" position - the head extended slightly backward, the neck flexed slightly forward and the chin lifted. In infants and children up to the age of 2 years, this may be facilitated by placing a small pillow or blanket under the torso.

        • In infants and children under the age of 2, flexion of the neck is unnecessary and the head should be placed on a flat surface with the chin lifted into the sniffing position[12]

    c. If cervical spine injury is suspected, endotracheal intubation is performed while maintaining manual in-line stabilization of the head and neck.

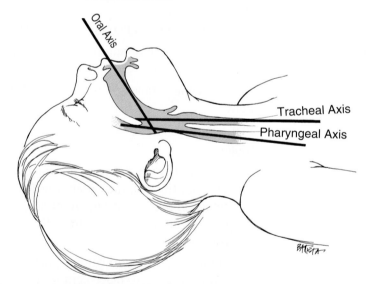

Figure 3-17. The axes of the mouth, pharynx and trachea aligned for endotracheal intubation.

6. Cricoid pressure (Sellick maneuver) may be applied to:

    • Aid placement of the ET tube into the tracheal opening through better visualization of the cords

    • Occlude the esophagus to minimize gastric distention and risk of aspiration

7. Cease ventilation of the patient (begin timing)*

With the laryngoscope held in the LEFT hand:

   a. Insert the blade into the right side of the mouth, sweeping the tongue to the left

   b. Do not use a prying motion or use the teeth as a fulcrum - pull up and away

   c. Visualize the epiglottis, then the vocal cords

   d. Insert the endotracheal tube from the right corner of the mouth

   e. Advance the endotracheal tube until the vocal cord marker on the endotracheal tube is at the level of the vocal cords

      • If a cuffed endotracheal tube is used, inflate the cuff

   f. Holding the tube firmly with your thumb and index finger next to the patient's lips, ventilate the patient by attaching the bag-valve device to the endotracheal tube

(End timing)

*Time should not exceed 30 seconds

Confirm Tube Placement

1. Observe the chest for symmetrical movement with ventilation

2. Auscultate

   a. Listen over each lateral chest wall, high in axillae, for equal breath sounds

   b. Listen over the stomach

      • Breath sounds may be heard over the stomach in infants but should not be louder than midaxillary sounds

3. Fogging of or condensation in the endotracheal tube is not a reliable indicator of endotracheal intubation

4. Note the end-tidal carbon dioxide level, if available.

5. Ultimate confirmation of proper endotracheal tube placement should be obtained by chest x-ray because:

   a. Right mainstem bronchus intubation is more likely in the child than in the adult due to the relatively short trachea of the infant and young child

      • The carina is the point where the trachea bifurcates into the right and left mainstem bronchi

   b. Breath sounds may be transmitted from the esophagus to the lung fields

6. Once proper tube position is confirmed, note the cm marking on the endotracheal tube at the level of the patient's lips. This will assist in noting accidental displacement of the endotracheal tube.

Signs of Proper Endotracheal Tube Placement

1. Symmetrical chest rise with positive pressure ventilation
2. Presence of bilateral equal breath sounds
3. Improvement in heart rate, color, blood pressure and perfusion
4. Absence of gurgling sounds over the stomach with positive-pressure ventilation
5. Direct visualization of the vocal cords during intubation

Securing the Endotracheal Tube

1. Note the cm markings on the endotracheal tube at the level of the patient's lips
2. Tear a piece of adhesive tape into the shape of a Y.
3. Wrap the torn piece of tape around the endotracheal tube, securing the intact portion of the tape to the maxilla.
    -   Securing the endotracheal tube to the movable mandible may result in displacement of the tube.
4. Fold the end of the tape for ease of later removal.
5. Recheck the cm markings on the endotracheal tube to be sure the tube was not dislodged.
6. Confirm tube position by chest x-ray.
7. Auscultate frequently to reevaluate the position of the endotracheal tube.

Complications

1. Aspiration
2. Bradycardia
3. Equipment failure
4. Tension pneumothorax
5. Inadvertent esophageal intubation
6. Dislodgement of the endotracheal tube
7. Inadvertent right mainstem bronchus intubation
8. Hypoxia due to prolonged or unsuccessful intubation
9. Obstruction of the endotracheal tube (mucus plug)
10. Trauma to the lips, teeth, tongue or soft tissues of the oropharynx.

Special Considerations

1. If breath sounds are absent bilaterally after intubation and gurgling is heard over the epigastrium, assume esophageal intubation.
    -   Remove the endotracheal tube and hyperventilate before reattempting intubation (if a cuffed endotracheal tube was used, deflate the cuff before removal).

2. If breath sounds are diminished on the left after intubation but present on the right, assume right mainstem bronchus intubation.
   - Pull back the endotracheal tube slightly and reevaluate breath sounds (if a cuffed endotracheal tube was used, deflate the cuff, pull back the tube slightly, reinflate the cuff and reevaluate breath sounds).

3. If proper endotracheal tube position has been confirmed but inadequate lung expansion occurs, check the following:
   a. Bag-valve device leak
      - Use a different bag or
      - Disconnect the bag-valve device from the endotracheal tube and occlude the endotracheal tube connection. Compress the bag to determine the site of the leak.
   b. The person ventilating is delivering too shallow a breath (short, rapid ventilations deliver an insufficient volume of air). Correct by delivering a larger breath.
   c. The pop-off valve on the bag-valve device is not depressed.
      - To properly ventilate patients with poor lung compliance, as in pulmonary edema or victims of near-drowning, higher than usual airway pressures are often needed
      - Pop-off valves may prevent generation of sufficient peak airway pressure to overcome the increase in airway resistance
   d. The endotracheal tube is too small and a large air leak is present.
      - If an uncuffed endotracheal tube was used, replace with a larger tube.
      - If a cuffed endotracheal tube was used, the cuff should be inflated until the air leak disappears, using the minimum volume of air necessary.

4. Vital signs should be monitored before, during and after this procedure.
   a. Infants and young children are very sensitive to vagal stimulation which may occur as a result of stimulation of the posterior pharynx, larynx or trachea.

      b.   Interrupt the procedure and ventilate the patient with 100% oxygen via a bag-mask device if bradycardia occurs or the child's color or perfusion deteriorates.

- Heart rate < 80 beats/minute in the infant
- Heart rate < 60 beats/minute in the child

5.   Should take no more than 30 seconds for the procedure
6.   Should be performed only by trained personnel

Table 3-3. Suggested Sizes for Endotracheal Tubes and Suction Catheters.

SUGGESTED SIZES FOR ENDOTRACHEAL TUBES AND SUCTION CATHETERS

AGE	Internal Diameter of Tube, mm	Distance midtrachea to teeth/gums	Suction Catheters
Premature infant	2.5, 3.0 uncuffed	8 cm	5–6F
Term Infant	3.0, 3.5 uncuffed	9–10 cm	6–8F
6 mo	3.5, 4.0 uncuffed	10 cm	8F
1 year	4.0, 4.5 uncuffed	11 cm	8F
2 years	4.5, 5.0 uncuffed	12 cm	8F
4 years	5.0, 5.5 uncuffed	14 cm	10F
6 years	5.5 uncuffed	15 cm	10F
8 years	6.0 cuffed or uncuffed	16 cm	10F
10 years	6.5 cuffed or uncuffed	17 cm	12F
12 years	7.0 cuffed	18 cm	12F
Adolescent	7.0, 8.0 cuffed	20 cm	12F

Source: Chameides L, Hazinski MF (ed.): *Textbook of Pediatric Advanced Life Support.* Dallas: American Heart Association, 1994.

PERCUTANEOUS NEEDLE CRICOTHYROTOMY

Description   Method of providing ventilation by insertion of a large-bore over-the-needle catheter into the cricothyroid membrane with intermittent jet ventilation
- Temporary procedure

Indications   Upper airway obstruction that *cannot be relieved by other methods* including:

a. Head positioning

b. Suctioning

c. Foreign body airway maneuvers

d. Bag-valve mask ventilation

e. Endotracheal intubation

Obstruction may be due to:
- Foreign body
- Fracture of the larynx
- Severe orofacial injuries
- Severe oropharyngeal hemorrhage
- Infection

Advantages   Allows rapid entrance to the airway for temporary ventilation and oxygenation

Disadvantages
1. Does not allow for direct suctioning of secretions
2. Does not allow for efficient elimination of carbon dioxide
3. Invasive procedure
4. Requires skilled rescuers to perform with frequent retraining

Equipment
1. Gloves, goggles
2. Oxygen source
3. Bag-valve device (size appropriate for patient)
4. 14 gauge over-the-needle catheter
5. 10 ml syringe
6. 3.0 mm endotracheal tube adaptor
7. Suction equipment
8. Adhesive tape

Procedure
1. Body substance isolation precautions
2. Place the patient in a supine position
3. Identify landmarks
   - Thyroid cartilage
   - Cricoid cartilage
   - Cricothyroid membrane
4. Cleanse the site

5. Using a large-bore cannula (at least 14-guage) carefully puncture the skin in the midline directly over the cricothyroid membrane
6. Direct the needle and syringe caudally and posteriorly at a 45-degree angle
7. Carefully insert the needle and catheter through the cricothyroid membrane, maintaining negative pressure as the needle is advanced
    *   Aspiration of air signifies entry in the tracheal lumen
8. Advance the catheter over the needle until the catheter hub is flush with the skin
    *   Hold the catheter hub in place to prevent displacement while removing the needle and syringe
9. Attach transtracheal ventilation system tubing to the catheter and ventilate
    *   Or, the catheter may be connected to a 3 mm endotracheal tube adaptor and attached to a bag-valve device connected to an oxygen source
10. Observe rise and fall of the chest and auscultate for adequate ventilation
11. Secure the catheter in place

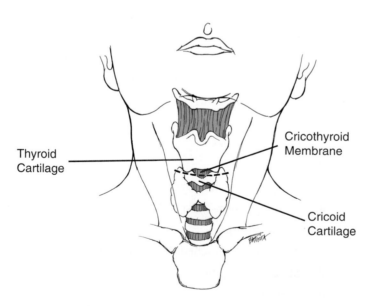

Figure 3-18. Anatomical landmarks for cricothyrotomy.

Complications

1. Bleeding
2. Infection
3. Hematoma
4. Hypoxemia
5. Catheter dislodgement
6. Subcutaneous emphysema
7. Esophageal perforation if needle advanced too far

NEEDLE THORACOSTOMY

Description Insertion of an over-the-needle catheter into the chest to relieve a tension pneumothorax

Indications Suspected tension pneumothorax as evidenced by:

- Decreasing level of consciousness
- Severe respiratory distress
- Tracheal deviation away from the affected side
- Hypotension
- Hyperresonance to percussion and diminished breath sounds on the affected side

Equipment Gloves

Over-the-needle catheter (18- to 20-guage)

Syringe

Intravenous extension tubing

Small bottle of sterile water

Procedure

1. Body substance isolation precautions
2. Identify landmarks - the second intercostal space at the midclavicular line
3. Cleanse the skin
4. Insert the needle perpendicular to the skin just over the third rib into the intercostal space on the affected side, midclavicular line.
5. Draw back the plunger of the syringe and then release it.
   a. If the plunger does not move, there is air in the syringe.
      - Remove the needle, leaving the catheter in place
      - Connect one end of the IV extension tubing to the catheter and place the other end in a small bottle of sterile water
   b. If the plunger is drawn back into the base of the syringe, no air is present.
      - Remove the needle
      - Repeat the procedure on the opposite hemithorax[13]

6. Reassess breath sounds and respiratory status.
   - Heart rate, blood pressure and perfusion should rapidly return to normal if decompression was successful.
7. Secure the catheter to prevent dislodgement.

Complications
1. Pneumothorax
2. Pleural infection
3. Laceration of the lung
4. Laceration of the intercostal vessel(s) with resultant hemorrhage

NONINVASIVE RESPIRATORY MONITORING

PULSE OXIMETRY

Description and Function
1. A noninvasive method of continuously monitoring pulse rate, pulse amplitude and arterial oxygen saturation.
2. A sensor probe or clip is attached to the patient.
   a. The pulse oximeter measures the difference in intensity of two wavelengths of light (red and infrared) passing through the vascular bed.
   b. Oxygenated (saturated/red) hemoglobin absorbs and reflects light differently than deoxygenated (desaturated/blue) hemoglobin.
   c. The ratio of red to infrared absorption is calculated by the pulse oximeter to determine oxygen saturation.
3. Sensors are available in different sizes for the neonate, infant, pediatric and adult patient.

Uses
1. May provide an early indication of respiratory deterioration and development of hypoxemia.
2. Should be used during stabilization and transport

Limitations
The value of pulse oximetry may be limited in:
1. Hypothermia
2. Cardiac arrest
3. Carbon monoxide poisoning
4. Inadequate peripheral perfusion (shock)
5. Methemoglobinemia

END-TIDAL CO₂ MONITORING (CAPNOGRAPHY)

Description and Function	1. The end-tidal CO_2 detector is attached directly to (or between) an endotracheal tube between the ventilation device (bag-valve device, automatic transport ventilator or mechanical ventilator) and the tube.
	2. **Capnography** is a method of assessing ventilation by measuring end-tidal volume carbon dioxide ($PetCO_2$) concentrations in expired air.
Types	There are two main types of end-tidal CO_2 devices:

1. Electronic
    a. Those used in the hospital setting permit intermittent or continuous monitoring of carbon dioxide elimination.
    b. Some portable electronic units are useful for confirmation of endotracheal tube placement but do not display actual carbon dioxide concentration.
2. Colorimetric
    a. Plastic, inexpensive, disposable device that is placed between the ventilation device and the endotracheal tube.
    b. As exhaled gases pass through the device's pH-sensitive membrane, the tint of the color indicator changes. The color of the membrane is compared with a color chart that accompanies the device, estimating the end-tidal CO_2 concentration.

Uses	In the patient with a pulse and adequate blood pressure, an end-tidal CO_2 detector is of value in verifying endotracheal tube placement. A persistent, low value strongly suggests the endotracheal tube has been improperly placed in the esophagus.
Limitations	1. Should be used in infants larger than 2 kilograms
	2. Findings may be misleading due to low cardiac output in cardiac arrest.

Figure 3-19. Colorimetric end-tidal CO_2 detector.

REFERENCES

1. Eichelberger M. *Pediatric Emergencies: A Manual for Prehospital Care Providers,* Englewood Cliffs, Prentice-Hall, 1992.

2. Eichelberger, M. (ed.), *Pediatric Trauma: Prevention, Acute Care, Rehabilitation.* St. Louis: Mosby-Year Book, 1993.

3. Chameides L, Hazinski MF (ed.), *Textbook of Pediatric Advanced Life Support.* Dallas: American Heart Association, 1994, p. 4-7.

4. Fuhrman, B. *Pediatric Critical Care.* St. Louis: Mosby-Year Book, 1992.

5. Fuhrman, B. *Pediatric Critical Care.* St. Louis: Mosby-Year Book, 1992.

6. Chameides, L., Hazinski MF (ed.), *Textbook of Pediatric Advanced Life Support.* Dallas: American Heart Association, 1994, p. 4-9.

7. Bloom R (ed.), *Textbook of Neonatal Resuscitation.* Dallas: American Heart Association, 1994.

8. Chameides L, Hazinski MF (ed.), *Textbook of Pediatric Advanced Life Support.* Dallas: American Heart Association, 1994, p. 4-12.

9. Chameides L, Hazinski MF (ed.), *Textbook of Pediatric Advanced Life Support.* Dallas: American Heart Association, 1994, p. 4-12.

10. Flynn J. *Introduction to Critical Care Skills,* St. Louis, 1993, Mosby–Year Book.

11. Chameides L, Hazinski MF (ed.), *Textbook of Pediatric Advanced Life Support.* Dallas: American Heart Association, 1994, p. 4-13.

12. Chameides L, Hazinski MF (ed.), *Textbook of Pediatric Advanced Life Support.* Dallas: American Heart Association, 1994, p. 4-16.

13. Quan L, Seidel JS (ed.), *Instructor's Manual for Pediatric Advanced Life Support.* Dallas: American Heart Association, 1995, p. 2-13.

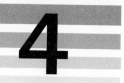

4 Vascular Access

OBJECTIVES

1. Describe the indications for vascular access.

2. Identify the preferred intravenous solutions for use in cardio-pulmonary arrest.

3. Describe the various types of intravenous cannulae.

4. List local complications of intravascular access.

5. List systemic complications of intravascular access.

6. Describe the advantages and disadvantages of peripheral veni-puncture.

7. Identify the most commonly used peripheral venipuncture sites in the pediatric patient.

8. State the indications for central venous access.

9. Describe the advantages and disadvantages of central venous access.

10. Describe complications of central venous catheter placement.

11. Describe the Seldinger technique for central venous catheter placement.

12. Identify the anatomical landmarks for femoral, internal jugular and subclavian vein cannulation.

13. State the indications for intraosseous infusion.

14. Identify the anatomical landmarks for intraosseous placement.

15. Describe alternatives to establishing venous access.

Indications for
Vascular Access

1. Delivery of medications

2. Administration of volume expanders

3. Obtain blood specimens for laboratory analysis

4. Administration of maintenance solutions

General Principles	1. If no IV exists prior to a cardiopulmonary arrest, the preferred access site is the largest, most easily accessible vein that does not interrupt resuscitative efforts.

2. If a central line is in place when an arrest occurs, it should be used for drug administration during the resuscitation effort.

3. The preferred IV solutions in cardiac arrest are normal saline or lactated Ringer's solution.
   - Large volumes of dextrose-containing solutions should not be infused because hyperglycemia may:
     - induce osmotic diuresis
     - produce or aggravate hyperkalemia
     - worsen ischemic brain injury

4. Medications administered via a peripheral vein during CPR should be followed with a saline flush of at least 5ml to facilitate delivery into the central circulation

TYPES OF IV CANNULAE

BUTTERFLY NEEDLES

Description

1. Short, metal needle with two plastic side arms (wings) with attached tubing
2. Available in 27 to 19 gauge sizes
3. Also referred to as scalp-vein needles

Advantages

1. May be used to obtain blood samples
2. Design (wings) facilitates insertion by providing a handle to grip
3. Wings allow the needle to be taped securely in place

Disadvantages

Tend to infiltrate easily, therefore this device should not be used for primary venous access during resuscitation efforts.

OVER-THE-NEEDLE CATHETERS

Description

1. A plastic or teflon catheter over a needle.
2. The needle within the catheter is used for the venipuncture. After venipuncture, the catheter is advanced into the vein and the needle removed.
3. The length of catheter is limited by the length of the needle
4. The puncture in the vein is the size of the catheter, which reduces the possibility of bleeding around the venipuncture site.
5. Available in 24 to 10 gauge sizes (22-24 gauge usually used for infants).

Advantages

1. More comfortable for the patient than the butterfly needle since the catheter is pliable.

2. Incidence of infiltration is lower because the blunt tip of the catheter reduces the chance of puncturing the vein.

3. May be used to cannulate the veins on the back of the hands, feet, and antecubital fossa as well as the external jugular, femoral and saphenous veins.

Disadvantages

Possibility of catheter-fragment embolism exists if proper insertion technique is not followed.

THROUGH-THE-NEEDLE CATHETERS

Description

1. Primary use is for administration of medications and fluids into the central circulation.

2. After the vein is entered with the needle, the catheter is inserted through the needle into the vein. A needle guard is placed over the tip of the needle to prevent the catheter from being sheared off by the needle after it is in place.

Advantages

Useful for accessing the central venous circulation when attempts to establish peripheral vascular access have proven futile.

Disadvantages

1. Risk of infection
   - The diameter of the puncture wound from the needle is larger than the catheter - provides a possible port of entry for organisms.

2. Risk of the sharp tip of the needle shearing off the end of the catheter, producing a catheter-fragment embolus
   - Never pull backward through the needle
   - If the catheter cannot be advanced through the needle, both the needle and catheter must be removed as a unit.

CATHETER-INTRODUCING SHEATH/DILATOR

Description

A guidewire (Seldinger technique) is used to introduce a dilator and sheath into the central venous circulation after initial venipuncture with a small-gauge needle or over-the-needle catheter.

After the dilator and sheath are passed over the guidewire into the vein, the guidewire and dilator are removed, leaving the sheath in place. The sheath may then be attached to an administration set for fluid administration.

COMPLICATIONS OF INTRAVASCULAR ACCESS

Local Complications
1. Cellulitis
2. Phlebitis
3. Thrombosis
4. Hematoma formation

Systemic Complications
1. Sepsis
2. Air embolism
3. Catheter-fragment embolism
4. Pulmonary thromboembolism

PERIPHERAL VENOUS ACCESS

Considerations

Infusion pumps should be used for all IV infusions in infants and children to avoid inadvertent circulatory overload unless large volumes of fluid are deliberately administered as part of the resuscitation effort.

Mini-drip infusion sets should be used and closely monitored if infusion pumps are not available.

Advantages
1. Effective route for fluid and medication administration
   - Medications administered during CPR should be followed with a saline flush to facilitate delivery into the central circulation
2. Does not require interruption of resuscitative efforts
3. Easier to learn than central venous access techniques
4. Results in fewer complications than central venous access

Disadvantages
1. In circulatory collapse, peripheral veins may be hard to locate
2. Small vessel diameter
3. Greater distance from the central circulation

Venipuncture Sites
1. Scalp veins (infants)
   a. Very small veins found close to the surface and more easily seen than extremity veins
   b. Rarely useful during resuscitation efforts
   c. May be useful for fluid administration and medication administration after patient stabilization

2. Upper extremity veins
    a. Forearm veins - may be difficult to locate in chubby babies
        Cephalic
        Median basilic
        Median antecubital
    b. Dorsal hand veins
        Tributaries of the cephalic and basilic veins
        Dorsal venous arch

3. Lower extremity veins
    a. Saphenous
    b. Median marginal
    c. Dorsal venous arch

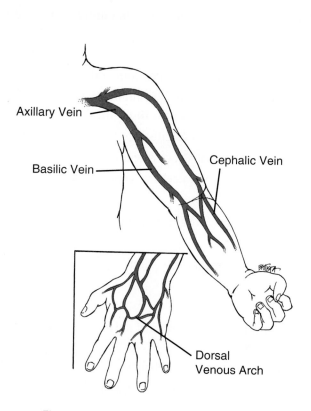

Figure 4-1. Veins of the forearm.

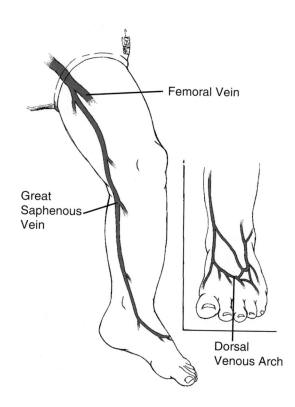

Figure 4-2. Lower extremity veins.

Procedure - Scalp Vein Cannulation

1. Body substance isolation precautions (gloves, goggles).
2. Assemble the necessary equipment.
3. Immobilize the patient.
4. Shave the site and surrounding skin if necessary.
5. Apply a tourniquet around the head (rubberband).
6. Cleanse the site.
7. Insert the needle through the skin and advance slowly into the vein (aiming toward the heart) until a flash of blood appears.
8. Remove the tourniquet and infuse a small amount of IV solution (by means of a syringe attached to the needle).
9. If the IV site is patent, secure with tape and attach the needle to a prepared IV infusion set (make sure no bubbles are present in the tubing prior to connection).

Procedure - Extremity Vein Cannulation

1. Body substance isolation precautions (gloves, goggles).
2. Assemble the necessary equipment.
3. Immobilize the patient and the selected extremity.
4. Apply a venous tourniquet proximal to the access site.
5. Cleanse the site.
6. Insert the cannula at a 30 to 45-degree angle through the skin. Once through the skin, adjust the angle of the cannula so that it is parallel to the skin and advance slowly into the vein until a flash of blood appears.
9. Remove the tourniquet and attach the catheter to a prepared IV infusion set (make sure no bubbles are present in the tubing prior to connection).
10. Tape securely in place.

VENOUS ACCESS ALTERNATIVES

Intraosseous infusion

Endotracheal administration

Central venous access (deemphasized)

"During CPR in children 6 years of age or younger, intraosseous access should be established if reliable venous access cannot be achieved within three attempts or 90 seconds, whichever comes first."

"Intravenous or intraosseous drug administration is preferable to endotracheal durg administration. However, if it is expected that vascular access will not be achieved within 3-5 minutes, epinephrine should be administered by the endotracheal route."[1]

CENTRAL VENOUS ACCESS

Indications
1. Emergency access to venous circulation for administration of fluids and/or medications.

2. Central venous pressure measurement.

3. Administration of blood products.

4. Administration of parenteral hyperalimentation.

Advantages
1. Mechanism of delivery of rapid volume expansion

2. Delivery of medications closer to their sites of action

3. Ability to measure central venous pressure

Disadvantages
1. More training required than peripheral venipuncture

2. May interrupt resuscitation efforts

3. Higher complication rate than with peripheral venipuncture

Complications
1. Infection

2. Hemorrhage

3. Hemothorax

4. Air embolism

5. Pneumothorax

6. Cardiac tamponade

7. Catheter-fragment embolism

Sites
1. External jugular vein

2. Femoral vein

   • Preferred site for central venous access during resuscitation

   • Relatively easy to access

   • Cannulation usually does not interrupt resuscitation efforts

3. Internal jugular vein

4. Subclavian vein

   • Cannulated less frequently in the pediatric patient than in the adult

EXTERNAL JUGULAR VEIN

Anatomy

1. Lies superficially along the lateral portion of the neck

2. Extends from the angle of the mandible and passes downward until it enters the thorax at a point just above the middle of the clavicle and ends in the subclavian vein

Technique

1. Body substance isolation precautions (gloves, goggles)

2. Place the child in a supine, head-down position of 20-30-degrees

3. Restrain the child.

4. Turn the patient's head to the left (the right side is preferred for venipuncture), away from the venipuncture site.

5. Identify the external jugular vein.

6. Cleanse the venipuncture site. If time permits, anesthetize the site with 1% lidocaine.

7. For peripheral cannulation, insert an over-the-needle catheter into the vein. For central venous cannulation, insert a through-the-needle catheter or catheter-over-guidewire.

8. Advance the catheter until an adequate blood return is noted.

9. Make sure no bubbles are present in the tubing and attach an IV infusion set.

Considerations

1. Superficial and usually readily visible when the child is placed in a head-down position.

2. May not be readily accessible during resuscitation.

3. IV may be easily dislodged and positional with head movement.

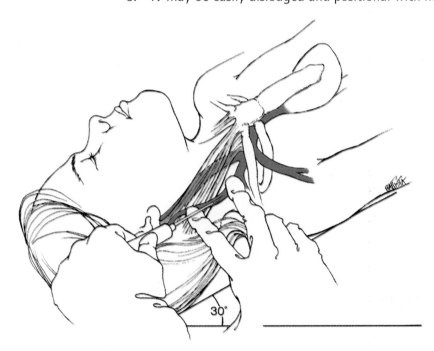

Figure 4-3. Cannulating the external jugular vein.

FEMORAL VEIN

Anatomy

1. The femoral vein lies directly medial to the femoral artery.
2. If a line is drawn between the anterior superior iliac spine and the symphysis pubis, the femoral artery runs directly across the mid-point - medial to that point is the femoral vein.
3. If the femoral artery pulse is palpable, the artery can be located with a finger and the femoral vein will lie immediately medial to the pulsation. A finger should remain on the artery to ease landmark identification and to avoid insertion of the catheter into the artery.

Technique

1. Body substance isolation precautions (gloves, goggles)
2. Restrain the lower extremities with slight external rotation.
3. Identify the femoral vein medial to the femoral artery.
4. Cleanse the site thoroughly. If time permits, anesthetize the area with 1% lidocaine.
5. Hold the catheter parallel to the vessel at a 15-30-degree angle to the horizontal.[2, 3]
6. Advance the catheter slowly until a free flow of blood is obtained.
7. Remove the needle, or guidewire and dilator, and secure the catheter.

Advantages

1. Relatively easy to access
2. Distant from major sites of activity during resuscitative efforts

Disadvantages

Long delivery time of drugs into the central circulation (due to pooling of fluids and medications in the inferior vena cava during external chest compressions) unless a long catheter with a tip that extends above the diaphragm is used

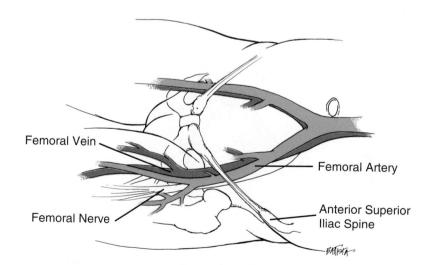

Femoral Vein

Femoral Artery

Femoral Nerve

Anterior Superior
Iliac Spine

Figure 4-4. Anatomy of the femoral vein.

INTERNAL JUGULAR VEIN

Anatomy

Runs from the base of the skull downward along the carotid artery until it enters the chest to meet with the subclavian vein behind the clavicle

Right side of the neck is preferred
- Dome of the right lung and pleura is lower than the left
- More or less a straight line to the right atrium
- Thoracic duct not in the way (empties on the left side)

Technique - Central (Middle) Approach

1. Body substance isolation precautions (gloves, goggles)
2. Place the child in a supine, head-down position of 20-45-degrees.
3. Restrain the child.
4. Turn the patient's head to the left (the right side is preferred for venipuncture), away from the venipuncture site.
5. Identify landmarks by observation and palpation (triangle formed by the two lower heads of the sternomastoid muscle and the clavicle).
6. Cleanse the venipuncture site. If time permits, anesthetize the site with 1% lidocaine.
7. Insert the catheter (attached to a syringe) at a 30-45-degree angle, while applying gentle pressure to the syringe, into the apex of the triangle aiming caudally and laterally toward the ipsilateral nipple.
8. When a free flow of blood enters the syringe, remove the syringe and occlude the needle hub with a gloved finger to prevent air embolism.
9. Advance the guidewire or catheter to the junction of the superior vena cava and right atrium during a positive-pressure breath or spontaneous exhalation.

    If a guidewire was used, remove the needle and pass a catheter or catheter-introducing sheath over the wire.
10. Secure the catheter or introducer in place. Make sure no bubbles are present in the tubing and attach an IV infusion set.
11. Verify catheter position via chest x-ray.

Considerations

1. Adjacent structures easily damage
2. More training required than with peripheral venipuncture
3. May interrupt resuscitative efforts
4. Higher complication rate than with peripheral venipuncture
5. Limits patient neck movement

SUBCLAVIAN VEIN

Anatomy

1. The subclavian vein is a continuation of the axillary vein, beginning at the point where this vein crosses over the first rib and under the medial half of the clavicle.

2. The subclavian is immobilized by small attachments to the first rib and clavicle.

3. The subclavian merges with the internal jugular vein to form the innominate (brachiocephalic) vein.

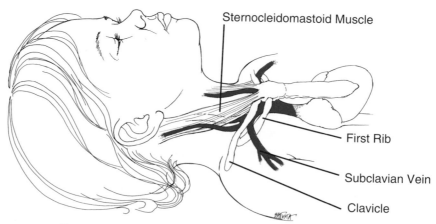

Figure 4-5. Anatomy of the subclavian vein.

Technique - Infraclavicular Approach

1. Body substance isolation precautions (gloves, goggles)

2. Place the child in a supine, head-down position of 20-30-degrees.

3. Restrain the child.

4. Identify landmarks - the junction of the middle and medial thirds of the clavicle.

5. Cleanse the venipuncture site. If time permits, anesthetize the site with 1% lidocaine.

6. Insert the needle (attached to a syringe) directed toward a fingertip placed in the suprasternal notch, just under the clavicle at the junction of the middle and medial thirds of the clavicle.

7. Slowly advance the needle while maintaining gentle suction on the plunger of the syringe.

8. When a free flow of blood enters the syringe, remove the syringe and occlude the needle hub with a gloved finger to prevent air embolism.

9. Advance the guidewire or catheter to the superior vena cava during a positive-pressure breath or spontaneous exhalation.

   • If a guidewire was used, remove the needle and pass a catheter or catheter-introducing sheath over the wire.

10. Secure the catheter or introducer in place. Make sure no bubbles are present in the tubing and attach an IV infusion set.

11. Verify catheter position via chest x-ray.

Considerations

1. Not recommended for small children unless alternate routes are not available.

2. Significant risk of pneumothorax, hemothorax, subclavian artery puncture.

3. More training required than with peripheral venipuncture

4. May interrupt CPR

5. Higher complication rate than with peripheral venipuncture.

INTRAOSSEOUS ACCESS

Considerations

1. The intraosseous site is not a site of first choice for vascular access.

2. Intraosseous cannulation is a temporary measure. Another form of vascular access should be sought once the child's condition is stabilized.

3. Medications should be followed with a saline flush of at least 5 ml to facilitate delivery into the central circulation.

Indications[4]

Child 6 years of age or younger when reliable venous access cannot be obtained within three attempts or 90 seconds, whichever comes first.

1. Multi-system trauma with associated shock and/or severe hypo-volemia

2. Severe dehydration associated with vascular collapse and/or loss of consciousness

3. Unresponsive and in need of immediate drug or fluid resuscitation
   a. Burns
   b. Status asthmaticus
   c. Sepsis
   d. Near-drowning
   e. Cardiac arrest
   f. Anaphylaxis

Contraindications

1. Pelvic fracture

2. Fracture in the extremity proximal to or in the bone selected for intraosseous access.

Equipment

1. Gloves, goggles
2. Betadine
3. Tape
4. 10 ml syringe
5. Sterile 4 x 4 gauze
6. IV solution
7. IV administration set
8. Kling (for stabilization after successful cannulation)
9. Pressure infusion bag or IV infusion pump
10. Rigid spinal needle with stylet, preferable a specifically designed intraosseous needle or Jamshidi-type bone marrow needle

Landmarks

The **preferred** site is the anteromedial (flat) surface of the proximal tibia, 1-3 cm (1 finger's width) below and just medial to the tibial tuberosity.

Other sites include:

1. Distal femur
   - Approximately 3 cm above the knee
2. Distal tibia
   - 1-3 cm above the medial malleolus on the surface of the tibia near the ankle
   - Believed by some to be the site of choice in older children due to the increased thickness of the proximal tibia compared to that of the distal tibia

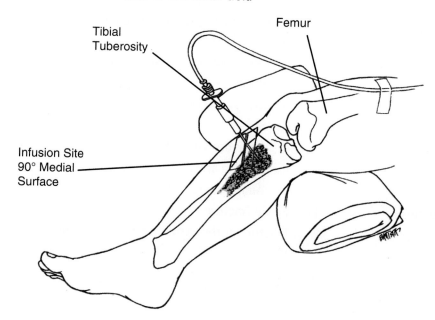

Figure 4-6. The preferred site for intraosseous infusion is the anteromedial (flat) surface of the proximal tibia, approximately one finger's width below and just medial to the tibial tuberosity.

Technique	1. Body substance isolation precautions (gloves, goggles).
	2. Place the infant or child in a supine position and externally rotate the leg to display the medial aspect of the extremity.
	3. Identify the landmarks for needle insertion.
	4. Cleanse the puncture site.
	5. With the needle angled away from the joint, insert the needle using firm pressure and a twisting motion.
	a. Angling away from the joint reduces the likelihood of damage to the epiphyseal growth plate.
	b. Firm pressure pushes the needle through the skin and subcutaneous tissue. A twisting motion is necessary to advance the needle through the periosteum of the bone.
	6. Advance the needle until a sudden decrease in resistance ("pop") is felt as the needle enters the marrow cavity.
	7. Remove the stylet.
	8. Attach a 10 ml syringe and aspirate.*
	a. "If the needle is properly placed in the bone marrow, aspiration of blood with marrow may be possible, but does not always occur."[5]
	*Aspiration may cause the needle to become obstructed with marrow, bone fragments or tissue
	b. Other indicators of correct needle position include:
	• Fluid flows freely
	• Absence of signs of significant subcutaneous infiltration
	• The needle stands upright without support
	9. Remove the syringe and attach the IV tubing - a pressure infuser bag or IV infusion pump may be needed to infuse fluids.
	10. Secure the needle with tape.
Complications	1. Extravasation
	2. Tibial fracture
	3. Osteomyelitis
	4. Epiphyseal injury
	5. Lower extremity compartment syndrome
	6. Loss of vascular access site may occur due to needle obstruction by marrow, bone fragments, or tissue

REFERENCES

1. Chameides L, Hazinski MF (ed.), *Textbook of Pediatric Advanced Life Support.* Dallas: American Heart Association, 1994, p. 5-2.

2. Barkin, R. (ed.), *Pediatric Emergency Medicine.* St. Louis: Mosby-Year Book, 1992.

3. Fuhrman, B. *Pediatric Critical Care.* St. Louis: Mosby-Year Book, 1992.

4. Allison, E. (ed.), *Advanced Life Support Skills.* St. Louis: Mosby-Year Book, 1994.

5. Eichelberger M. *Pediatric Emergencies: A Manual for Prehospital Care Providers,* Englewood Cliffs, Prentice-Hall, 1992.

QUIZ – AIRWAY MANAGEMENT AND VASCULAR ACCESS

1. Endotracheal intubation:

    a. is contraindicated in the unresponsive patient
    b. eliminates the risk of aspiration of gastric contents
    c. should be preceded by efforts to ventilate by another method
    d. when attempted, should be performed in less than 60 seconds

2. Advantages of peripheral venous access include:

    1. Does not require interruption of resuscitative efforts
    2. Small vessel diameter
    3. Easy technique to learn
    4. Short distance from the central circulation
    5. Effective route for medication administration

    a. 2, 3
    b. 2, 4, 5
    c. 1, 3, 5
    d. 1, 4, 5

3. The maximum length of time for suctioning the pediatric patient is:

    a. 5 seconds
    b. 10 seconds
    c. 15 seconds
    d. 30 seconds

4. Which of the following is not a vein of the upper extremity that may be used for intravenous access?

    a. cephalic
    b. median basilic
    c. median marginal
    d. median antecubital

5. A device useful for removal of thick secretions and particulate matter from the pharynx is the:

    a. face tent
    b. oropharyngeal airway
    c. rigid plastic suction device (tonsil-tip)
    d. flexible plastic suction catheter (whistle-tip)

6. Where is the femoral vein located relative to the femoral artery?

    a. lateral
    b. medial
    c. anterior
    d. posterior

7. If the heart rate drops to less than __ beats per minute in an infant or child during an intubation attempt, the procedure should be interrupted and the patient ventilated with 100% oxygen.

    a. 60
    b. 80
    c. 100
    d. 120

8. The preferred site for intraosseous infusion in the child under the age of 6 years is the:

    a. sternum
    b. distal femur
    c. medial malleolus
    d. anteromedial aspect of the tibia

9. Stridor is:

    a. a high-pitched inspiratory sound associated with upper airway obstruction
    b. a bluish discoloration of the skin and mucous membranes from lack of oxygen
    c. a crackling sound caused by air entering the alveoli of the lungs that have a buildup of fluid
    d. a visible sinking-in of the soft tissues of the chest between the ribs associated with increased breathing effort

10. The suggested size endotracheal tube for a 2 year old would be:

    a. 3.5 mm I.D.
    b. 4.0 mm I.D.
    c. 4.5 mm I.D.
    d. 5.5 mm I.D.

11. Medications delivered by the peripheral venous or intraosseous route should be followed by a saline flush of at least ____ to facilitate delivery to the central circulation.

    a. 5 ml
    b. 10 ml
    c. 20 ml
    d. 30 ml

12. When tracheal suctioning is performed, suction is applied:

    a. only during insertion of the catheter
    b. only during withdrawal of the catheter
    c. during insertion and removal of the catheter
    d. it makes no difference when suction is applied

13. A seven year old is found unresponsive. Describe how you will insert an oropharyngeal airway in this patient.

_____

_____

14. A short, metal needle with two plastic side arms with attached tubing best describes a(n):

   a. butterfly needle
   b. dilator sheath assembly
   c. over-the-needle-catheter
   d. through-the-needle-catheter

15. The name given the technique of applying cricoid pressure during endotracheal intubation is:

   a. Vagal maneuver
   b. Sellick maneuver
   c. Heimlich maneuver
   d. Seldinger maneuver

16. Indicate the equation that may be used to estimate endotracheal tube size for children over the age of one year.

_____

17. Indicators of correct intraosseous needle position include:

   1. Fluids flow freely
   2. Absence of signs of significant subcutaneous infiltration
   3. Needle stands upright without support
   4. Bone marrow is aspirated

   a. 1, 4
   b. 2, 3
   c. 1, 2, 3
   d. 1, 2, 3, 4

18. An infant has been intubated. Describe how you will confirm placement of the endotracheal tube.

_____

_____

19. A 6 year old male with a history of asthma experienced a sudden onset of difficulty breathing during a soccer game. Initial examination reveals the airway to be clear and chest rise to be symmetrical. Auscultation reveals bilaterally diminished breath sounds with expiratory wheezes. Nasal flaring is evident. The patient is diaphoretic and lethargic. During the course of your examination the child becomes cyanotic and apneic. A pulse is present at 84 beats per minute.

Describe your initial management of this patient.

_____

_____

20. Which of the following are correct regarding vascular access?

1. If a central line is in place when an arrest occurs, it should be used for drug administration during the resuscitation effort.
2. The preferred IV solution in cardiac arrest is 5% dextrose in water.
3. In children 6 years of age or younger, if reliable venous access cannot be achieved within three attempts or 90 seconds (whichever comes first), alternative routes for medication administration must be considered.
4. Infusion pumps should be used for IV infusions in infants and children to avoid inadvertent circulatory overload.

    a. 1, 2, 3
    b. 1, 2, 4
    c. 1, 3, 4
    d. 2, 3, 4

QUIZ ANSWERS – AIRWAY MANAGEMENT AND VASCULAR ACCESS

QUESTION	ANSWER	RATIONALE	STUDY GUIDE PAGE REFERENCE	PALS PAGE REFERENCE
1	C	Endotracheal (ET) intubation should be preceded by attempts to ventilate by another method. ET intubation reduces, but does not eliminate, the risk of aspiration of gastric contents. When attempted, ET intubation should be performed in less than 30 seconds.	98, 102	4-14
2	C	Advantages of peripheral venous access include: effective route for medication administration, does not require interruption of resuscitative efforts, easier to learn than central venous access, results in fewer complications than central venous access.	117	N/A
3	A	The maximum length of time for suctioning the pediatric patient is 5 seconds.	92	4-8
4	C	Veins of the upper extremity that may be used for intravenous access include the cephalic, median basilic and median antecubital. The median marginal vein is located in the lower extremity.	118	5-3
5	C	The rigid plastic suction device (tonsil-tip, Yankauer) is useful for removal of thick secretions and particulate matter from the pharynx.	92	4-7
6	B	The femoral vein is medial to the femoral artery.	122	5-9
7	A	If the heart rate drops to less than 60 beats per minute in the infant or child, or a heart rate consistently below the patient's baseline, the procedure should be interrupted and the patient ventilated with 100% oxygen.	106	4-15

8	D	In children under the age of 6 years, the preferred intraosseous infusion site is the anteromedial aspect of the tibia.	126	5-6
9	A	Stridor is a high-pitched inspiratory sound indicative of upper airway obstruction. (B) describes cyanosis. (C) describes rales. (D) describes retractions.	49	2-3
10	C	The suggested endotracheal tube size for a 2 year old would be 4.5 mm I.D. (uncuffed). Although endotracheal tube size is more reliably based on the size of the patient than age (the use of a resuscitation tape may be helpful), tube size may be determined by use of the formula: [age (years)/4] + 4 or 16 + patient's age in years/4.	99, 106	4-15
11	A	Medications administered by the peripheral venous or intraosseous routes should be followed with a saline flush of at least 5 ml to facilitate delivery into the central circulation.	115	5-6, 6-5
12	B	Tracheal suction should be applied, using a rotating motion, only upon withdrawal of the catheter. Suctioning should be preceded and followed by a short period of ventilation with 100% oxygen.	92	4-8
13		Proper size is determined by aligning the airway on the side of the patient's face and selecting an airway that extends from the corner of the mouth to the angle of the jaw. The airway should be inserted using a tongue blade to depress the tongue. If a tongue depressor is not available, the airway may be inverted for insertion into the mouth and rotated 180° into proper position as the airway approaches the back of the oropharynx (check local protocol).	89	4-7

14	A	A butterfly needle is a short, metal needle with two plastic side arms (wings) with attached tubing. Although this type of needle may be useful obtaining blood specimens, it should not be used for primary venous access during CPR due to the frequency with which infiltration occurs with this type of device.	115	5-3
15	B	The Sellick maneuver is the name given the technique of applying cricoid pressure during endotracheal intubation. This technique may also be used to help minimize gastric distention and aspiration during assisted ventilation.	102	4-11, 4-17
16		The equation [age (years)/4] + 4 may be used to estimate endotracheal tube size for children over the age of one year. Endotracheal tube size is more reliably based on patient size than age.	99	4-14
17	D	Indicators of correct intraosseous needle position include fluids flow freely, bone marrow is aspirated, absence of signs of significant subcutaneous infiltration, lack of resistance after the needle passes through the bony cortex, and the needle stands upright without support.	127	5-6
18		Proper endotracheal tube placement must be confirmed by: 1. Observing the chest for symmetrical movement 2. Auscultate for equal breath sounds over each lateral chest, high in the axillae 3. Confirmation of absent breath sounds over the stomach 4. Notation of the end-tidal carbon dioxide level (if available)	103	4-17

| 19 | | This child is exhibiting signs of probable respiratory failure as evidenced by diminished breath sounds and a decreased level of consciousness. Management efforts should include:
1. Separate the child from the caregiver
2. Control the airway-position the head
3. Administer 100% oxygen and assist ventilation with a bag-valve device. Intubate if the patient requires continuous bagging to maintain color. Confirm tube placement and secure in place.
4. Give nothing by mouth
5. Monitor pulse oximetry
6. Cardiac monitor
7. Establish vascular access | 44, 53 | 2-7 |
| 20 | C | The preferred IV solutions in cardiac arrest are normal saline or lactated Ringer's solution. 5% dextrose in water should not be used during resuscitation because hyperglycemia may induce osmotic diuresis, produce or aggravate hypokalemia, and worsen ischemic brain injury. Infusion pumps should be used for all IV infusions in infants and children to avoid inadvertent circulatory overload unless large volumes of fluid are deliberately administered as part of the resuscitation effort. | 114 | 6-2, 6-10 |

Fluids and Medications 5

Upon completion of this chapter, you will be able to:

1. Describe the location and effects of stimulation of alpha, beta and dopaminergic receptors.

2. Define the following terms:
   - Agonist
   - Antagonist
   - Chronotrope
   - Dromotrope
   - Inotrope
   - Parasympatholytic
   - Sympathomimetic

3. Identify the assessment parameters used to evaluate a child's response to fluid therapy.

4. Describe the technique for administration of medications via the endotracheal route.

5. Identify the mechanism of action, indications, dosage and precautions for each of the following medications:
   - Oxygen
   - Epinephrine
   - Calcium chloride
   - Glucose
   - Sodium bicarbonate
   - Adenosine
   - Lidocaine
   - Bretylium
   - Atropine
   - Dopamine
   - Dobutamine

Table 5-1. Review of the Autonomic Nervous System.

	SYMPATHETIC DIVISION	PARASYMPATHETIC DIVISION
RECEPTORS	**Alpha (œ)-1** • Located in vascular smooth muscle • Stimulation results in vasoconstriction **Alpha (œ)-2** • Located in the skeletal blood vessels • Inhibits the release of norepinephrine **Beta (ß)-1 (one heart)** • Located in the heart • Stimulation results in increased heart rate, increased conduction, increased contractility **Beta (ß)-2 (two lungs)** • Located in the smooth muscle of the bronchi and the skeletal blood vessels • Stimulation results in relaxation of the bronchi and vasodilation **Dopaminergic** • Located in the coronary arteries, renal, mesenteric and visceral blood vessels • Stimulation results in dilation	**Nicotinic** receptors located in skeletal muscle. **Muscarinic** receptors located in smooth muscle. Organs and the effects of parasympathetic stimulation: Bronchi • Stimulation results in constriction, increased secretion Eye • Pupillary constriction Salivary glands • Increased salivation Heart • Decreased heart rate GI tract • Increased secretions, increased peristalsis
NEUROTRANSMITTER	Epinephrine, norepinephrine	Acetylcholine
SYNONYMOUS TERMS	Adrenergic, sympathomimetic, catecholamine, anticholinergic, parasympatholytic, cholinergic blocker	Cholinergic, parasympathomimetic, sympathetic blocker, cholinomimetic, sympatholytic, adrenergic blocker
OPPOSITE TERMS	Sympatholytic, antiadrenergic, sympathetic blocker, adrenergic blocker	Parasympatholytic, anticholinergic, cholinergic blocker, vagolytic

Table 5-2. Terminology

TERMINOLOGY	
Dromotrope	A substance that affects AV conduction velocity • Positive dromotrope = increases AV conduction velocity • Negative dromotrope = decreases AV conduction velocity
Chronotrope	A substance that affects heart rate • Positive chronotrope = increases heart rate • Negative chronotrope = decreases heart rate
Inotrope	A substance that affects myocardial contractility • Positive inotrope = increases force of contraction • Negative inotrope = decreases force of contraction
Agonist	A drug or substance that produces a predictable response (stimulates action)
Antagonist	An agent that exerts an opposite action to another (blocks action)

VOLUME EXPANSION

Crystalloid solutions – isotonic solutions which provide transient expansion of the intravascular volume

1. Examples
   a. Normal saline
      • Contains sodium chloride in water
      • Isotonic
   b. Ringer's lactate
      • Contains sodium chloride, potassium chloride, calcium chloride and sodium lactate in water
      • Isotonic
2. Advantages
   a. Inexpensive
   b. Readily available
   c. Free from allergic reactions
3. Disadvantages
   a. Effectively expand the interstitial space and correct sodium deficits but do not effectively expand the circulating volume
   b. Only 1/4 of the solution remains in the plasma; 4-5 times the volume deficit must be infused to restore plasma volume

Colloid solutions - draw water from the intracellular compartment and interstitial space to expand intravascular volume

1. Examples
    a. 5% albumin
    b. Dextran
    c. Hetastarch (Hespan)
    d. Fresh frozen plasma
2. Advantages
    *   More efficient than crystalloid solutions in rapidly expanding the intravascular compartment
3. Disadvantages
    a. Expensive
    b. Short shelf-life
    c. Potential for adverse reactions

Blood

1. Indicated for severe acute hemorrhage
2. May be helpful in septic and other forms of shock but is not a first-line volume expander

Fluid Therapy in Hypovolemic Shock

1. Administer a 20 ml/kg fluid bolus of crystalloid solution when vascular access is obtained.
2. Administer as quickly as possible (in less than 20 minutes).
3. Reassess the patient. If signs of decreased perfusion persist, administer an additional 20 ml/kg fluid bolus.
4. Succeeding fluid boluses may be either crystalloid or colloid and are administered based on the patient's response to fluid therapy.

A child in hypovolemic shock may require 40-60 ml/kg in the first hour of resuscitation. In septic shock, 60-80 ml/kg may be required during the first hour of therapy.[1]

Evaluation of Patient Response to Fluid Therapy

Evaluate the patient's response to fluid therapy:
1. Skin color and temperature
2. Volume and quality of peripheral pulses
3. Mental status
4. Heart rate
5. Urine output

Hypotension is a late and often sudden sign of cardiovascular decompensation.

MEDICATION ADMINISTRATION – GUIDELINES

Peripheral Intravenous
Access

1. Effective route for administration of blood, crystalloids, colloids and medications.
2. The intravenous line should be flushed with at least 5 ml of normal saline after medication administration to speed delivery to the central circulation.
3. Central venous access has been de-emphasized.

Intraosseous Infusion

1. Effective route for administration of blood, crystalloids, colloids and medications.
2. Should be attempted in children less than 6 years of age after three attempts at peripheral intravenous access or after 90 seconds have elapsed, whichever comes first.
3. The intravascular line should be flushed with at least 5 ml of normal saline, after medication administration to speed delivery to the central circulation.
4. Dosages for intraosseous administration are the same as for intravenous administration.

Endotracheal Drug
Administration

1. Lidocaine, epinephrine, atropine and naloxone (LEAN or LANE) may be administered endotracheally.
2. Optimal dosing via this route has not been determined.
   a. The recommended dose of epinephrine administered endotracheally is 10 times the IV dose. Lidocaine, atropine, and naloxone are administered at 2-3 times the IV dose.
   b. Procedure:[2]

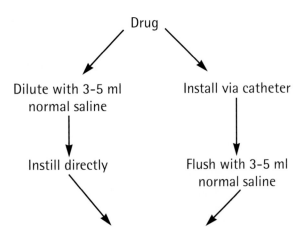

Drug

Dilute with 3-5 ml normal saline → Instill directly

Install via catheter → Flush with 3-5 ml normal saline

Deliver several forceful insufflations of the bag-valve device to enhance drug absorption

Intracardiac Injection

1. Epinephrine, atropine and sodium bicarbonate may be administered by cardiac injection.

2. Strongly discouraged due to hazards associated with the procedure including:

    a. Coronary laceration

    b. Cardiac tamponade

    c. Intractable dysrhythmias

    d. Interruption of chest compressions

The following pages provide a summary of medications that may be used in the management of the pediatric patient. The summary, presented in table format, is divided into the following categories:

Drugs Used for Cardiac Arrest and Resuscitation

Oxygen, Epinephrine, Calcium Chloride, Glucose, Sodium Bicarbonate

Drugs Used in the Treatment of Rhythm Disturbances

Treatment of SVT - Adenosine, Verapamil

Treatment of Bradycardia - Epinephrine, Atropine

Treatment of Ventricular Dysrhythmias - Lidocaine, Bretylium Tosylate

Drugs Used to Maintain Cardiac Output

Epinephrine, Dopamine, Dobutamine

Where possible, the American Heart Association's recommendations are based on the strength of supporting scientific evidence and are classified as follows:

Table 5-3. Classification of Therapeutic Interventions

Class I	Definitely helpful
Class IIa	Probably helpful
Class IIb	Possible helpful
Class III	Not indicated, may be harmful

DRUGS USED FOR CARDIAC ARREST AND RESUSCITATION

DRUG	MECHANISM OF ACTION/EFFECTS	INDICATIONS	DOSAGE	PRECAUTIONS
Oxygen	Increases oxygen tension Increases hemoglobin saturation of ventilation is supported Improves tissue oxygenation when circulation is maintained	1. All arrest situations 2. Suspected hypoxemia of any cause 3. Any condition of respiratory difficulty that may lead to cardiac arrest: • severe asthma • croup • epiglottitis • foreign body obstruction	In the spontaneously breathing patient: • Nasal cannula, simple face mask, blow-by In cardiac or respiratory arrest: positive-pressure ventilation with 100% oxygen	With prolonged administration of high flow oxygen, concern regarding toxic effects on the lungs and, in premature infants, on the eyes. *Do not withhold oxygen if signs of hypoxemia present.* Humidified oxygen helps prevent drying of the mucous membranes and loosens secretions.
Epinephrine **Trade Name:** Adrenalin **Classification:** Sympathomimetic, Natural Catecholamine	Produces beneficial effects in patients during cardiac arrest primarily because of its alpha-adrenergic stimulating properties Alpha-adrenergic effects: Increases peripheral vascular resistance (vasoconstriction) → increases diastolic pressure → increases myocardial and cerebral blood flow during CPR Beta-adrenergic effects: • Increased heart rate (+ chronotropy) • Increased myocardial contractility (+ inotropy) • Increased automaticity (+ dromotropy) • Results in increased myocardial oxygen consumption Most effective drug during resuscitation	Ventricular fibrillation Pulseless ventricular tachycardia Pulseless electrical activity Asystole	May be administered IV, IO, or ET **DOSING IN CARDIAC ARREST:** **Initial dose:** IV/IO: 0.01 mg/kg of 1:10,000 solution (0.1 ml/kg) ET: 0.1 mg/kg of 1:1000 solution (0.1 ml/kg) **Subsequent doses:** IV/IO/ET: 0.1 mg/kg of 1:1000 solution (0.1 ml/kg) IV/IO doses up to 0.2 mg/kg of 1:1000 solution may be effective May repeat every 3-5 minutes	• May cause local ischemia and ulceration if infiltration occurs • Epinephrine's actions are depressed by acidosis - adequate ventilation, circulation and correction of metabolic acidosis important • Alkaline solutions inactivate epinephrine • Dosing in arrest situations requires two different dilutions of epinephrine. Avoid errors in selection of concentration and dosing. • Endotracheal absorption is unpredictable. Once vascular access is obtained, administer IV. (Begin with the first IV dose–0.01 mg/kg of 1:10,000)

DRUG	MECHANISM OF ACTION/EFFECTS	INDICATIONS	DOSAGE	PRECAUTIONS
Calcium Chloride **Class:** Electrolyte	Increases myocardial contractile function	Probably helpful (Class IIa) in: • Documented hypocalcemia • Hyperkalemia • Hypermagnesemia • Calcium channel blocker overdose	May be administered IV or IO 20 mg/kg IV bolus of 10% solution—give slowly	• Bradycardia with rapid IV injection • Use with caution in digitalized patients - may precipitate severe dysrhythmias • Precipitates with sodium bicarbonate • Sclerosing to peripheral veins; extravasation may result in tissue sloughing
Glucose **Trade Name:** Dextrose **Class:** Carbohydrate	Main action is to replace glucose which is the principal source of energy for body cells. Because of its hypertonicity, it will also pull fluid into the intravascular space.	Class I (definitely helpful) in documented hypoglycemia	May be administered IV or IO 0.5-1.0 g/kg (2-4 ml/kg) of a 25% dextrose solution or 0.5-1.0 g/kg (5-10 ml/kg) of a 10% dextrose solution administered over 20 minutes	Extravasation can cause severe local tissue damage.
Naloxone **Trade Name:** Narcan **Class:** Narcotic Antagonist	Competes with opiod receptor sites in the central nervous system, displacing previously administered narcotic analgesics	Narcotic-induced respiratory depression	May be administered IV, IO, ET, IM, SQ If ≤5 years old or <20 kg: 0.1 mg/kg If >5 years old or >20 kg: 2.0 mg ET dose is 2-3 times IV dose	If half-life of naloxone is shorter than the half-life of the narcotic, it may be necessary to repeat the naloxone.
Sodium Bicarbonate **Class:** Alkalinizing Agent	Reacts with hydrogen ions to form carbonic acid (carbon dioxide and water) Produces paradoxical intracellular acidosis due to production of CO_2, which is freely diffusible into myocardial and cerebral cells and may depress function	Documented acidosis Prolonged arrest When serum alkalinization required • hyperkalemia • cyclic antidepressant overdose	May be administered IV or IO Initial dose: 1 mEq/kg Repeat dose: 0.5 mEq/kg every 10 minutes	• Should not be used until adequate ventilation is established • Sclerosing to small veins and produces chemical burns if extravasation occurs. • Incompatible with calcium and catecholamines. • Note: respiratory acidosis in cardiac arrest is best treated by administration of 100% oxygen and increasing the rate of ventilation.

DRUGS USED IN THE TREATMENT OF RHYTHM DISTURBANCES

TREATMENT OF SUPRAVENTRICULAR TACHYCARDIA (SVT)

DRUG	MECHANISM OF ACTION/EFFECTS	INDICATIONS	DOSAGE	PRECAUTIONS
Adenosine **Trade Name:** Adenocard **Class:** Endogenous Chemical, Antidysrhythmic	• Decreases sinus rate • Decreases conduction through the AV node • Can interrupt re-entrant pathways through the AV node • Has a direct effect on supraventricular tissue • Half-life is 5-10 seconds	Drug of choice for treatment of SVT. May be administered for unstable SVT before synchronized countershock if IV access is readily available.	May be administered **RAPID** IV or IO 0.1 mg/kg. If no effect, may increase to 0.2 mg/kg once Maximum single dose 12 mg	Temporary asystole may be observed for a few seconds. Side effects usually resolve spontaneously within 1-2 minutes due to short half-life. Contraindicated in: • Sick sinus syndrome • Second or third-degree AV block • Known hypersensitivity to the drug
Verapamil **Trade Name:** Isoptin, Calan **Class:** Calcium Channel Blocker	• Slows conduction and increases refractoriness in the AV node • May terminate reentrant dysrhythmias that require AV nodal conduction for their continuation • Decreases myocardial contractility • May exacerbate CHF in patients with severe left ventricular dysfunction	Not applicable	Not applicable	Should not be used to treat SVT in an emergency setting in infants less than 1 year of age, in children with CHF or myocardial depression, in children receiving beta-blockers or in those who have a bypass tract—profound bradycardia, hypotension, and asystole have been reported.[3]

TREATMENT OF BRADYCARDIA

DRUG	MECHANISM OF ACTION/EFFECTS	INDICATIONS	DOSAGE	PRECAUTIONS
Epinephrine **Trade Name:** Adrenalin **Classification** Sympathomimetic Natural Catecholamine	Beta-adrenergic effects: • Increased heart rate (+ chronotropy) • Increased myocardial contractility (+ inotropy) • Increased automaticity (+ dromotropy) • Results in increased myocardial oxygen consumption	Symptomatic brady-cardia unresponsive to ventilation and oxygen administration	IV/IO: 0.01 mg/kg of 1:10,000 solution (0.1 ml/kg) ET: 0.1 mg/kg of 1:1000 solution (0.1 ml/kg) Repeat every 3–5 minutes at the same dose	May cause tachycardia and produce ventricular ectopy. May cause local ischemia and ulceration if infiltration occurs.
Atropine Sulfate **Class:** Anticholinergic (Parasympathetic blocker)	Parasympathetic *blocking* (vagolytic) action: • Increases heart rate (accelerates sinus or atrial pacemakers) • Improves AV conduction	Class I (definitely helpful) in: • Symptomatic brady-cardia with AV block (uncommon event) • Vagally mediated bradycardia during intubation attempts Class IIb (possibly helpful) in: • Bradycardia with poor perfusion and hypotension (epi-nephrine first-line drug) • Asystole	May be administered **IV, IO, ET** 0.02 mg/kg (minimum dose 0.1 mg) Maximum single dose: 0.5 mg in child 1.0 mg in adolescent May be repeated in 5 minutes to a maximum total dose of 1.0 mg in child, 2.0 mg in adolescent Endotracheal dose is 2–3 times IV dose.	• Should be used to treat bradycardia only after adequate oxygenation and ventilation have been ensured since hypoxia is a common cause of bradycardia.[4] • Should not be pushed in doses of less than 0.1 mg as a paradoxical bradycardia may occur. • Administration of atropine may mask hypoxemia-induced bradycardia. Monitor oxygen saturation during intubation attempts with pulse oximetry and avoid prolonged intubation attempts.

TREATMENT OF VENTRICULAR DYSRHYTHMIAS

DRUG	MECHANISM OF ACTION/EFFECTS	INDICATIONS	DOSAGE	PRECAUTIONS
Lidocaine Hydrochloride **Trade Name** Xylocaine **Class** Ventricular Antidysrhythmic	Suppresses ventricular ectopy Raises the ventricular fibrillation threshold	Pulseless ventricular tachycardia or ventricular fibrillation that persists after defibrillation and administration of epinephrine Ventricular tachycardia with a pulse (may be administered before synchronized countershock *if* IV access has been achieved and lidocaine is readily available) Significant ventricular ectopy of unknown origin following resuscitation	May be administered IV, IO or ET 1 mg/kg (over 1-2 minutes in the patient with a pulse). Continuous infusion: 20-50 mcg/kg/min To prepare infusion: 60 x body weight in kilograms = # of mg of lidocaine to be added to a solution with a total volume of 100 ml (60 x kg = mg) Then: 1 ml/hr = 10 mcg/kg/min 2 ml/hr = 20 mcg/kg/min 5 ml/hr = 50 mcg/kg/min Endotracheal dose is 2-3 times the IV dose	Indications of toxicity are usually CNS related: • drowsiness • disorientation • muscle twitching • seizures Because lidocaine is metabolized in the liver, the maintenance infusion rate should not exceed 20 mcg/kg/min in: • patients with known liver disease, decreased cardiac output (CHF, shock) • cardiac arrest Contraindicated in children with wide-complex ventricular escape beats associated with bradycardia.
Bretylium Tosylate **Trade Name** Bretylol **Class** Ventricular Antidysrhythmic, Adrenergic Blocker	• Suppresses ventricular ectopy • Raises ventricular fibrillation threshold	Not a first-line antidysrhythmic Class IIb (possibly helpful) after defibrillation, epinephrine and lidocaine have failed to convert ventricular fibrillation or pulseless ventricular tachycardia	May be administered IV or IO **Refractory VF/pulseless VT:** 5 mg/kg rapid IV **bolus** followed by defibrillation. If VF persists, dose may be increased to 10 mg/kg and followed by defibrillation.	Additive effects with sympathomimetics No published facts on usefulness in pediatric patients

DRUGS USED TO MAINTAIN CARDIAC OUTPUT

DRUG	MECHANISM OF ACTION/EFFECTS	INDICATIONS	DOSAGE	PRECAUTIONS
Epinephrine **Trade Name:** Adrenalin **Class** Sympathomimetic Natural Catecholamine	Low-dose infusions (< 0.3 mcg/kg/min) generally produce predominate beta-adrenergic effects: • Increased heart rate (+ chronotropy) • Increased myocardial contractility (+ inotropy) • Increased automaticity (+ dromotropy) Higher dose infusions result in alpha-adrenergic effects: Increased peripheral vascular resistance (vasoconstriction), Increased pulse pressure Results in increased myocardial oxygen consumption	Treatment of shock with diminished systemic perfusion from any cause unresponsive to fluid resuscitation Poor perfusion following the restoration of a stable rhythm	Initial: 0.1 mcg/kg/min Titrate according to patient response up to 1.0 mcg/kg/min Higher infusion rates may be used during CPR (0.1-1.0 mcg/kg/min) To prepare infusion: 0.6 x body weight in kilograms = # of mg of epinephrine to be added to a solution for a total volume of 100 ml (0.6 x kg = mg) Then: 1 ml/hr = 0.1 mcg/kg/min 2 ml/hr = 0.2 mcg/kg/min	• May cause local ischemia and ulceration if extravasation occurs. • May cause tachycardia or ventricular ectopy. • High doses may produce excessive vasoconstriction, compromising blood flow to the extremities, kidneys and mesentery. • Do not discontinue abruptly - taper gradually. • Administer via an infusion pump.
Dopamine **Trade Name:** Intropin, Dopastat **Class:** Sympathomimetic Natural Catecholamine	Precursor of epinephrine that has dopaminergic, alpha and beta-adrenergic receptor stimulating actions Dose-related effects: Low dose (2.5 mcg/kg/min): • Dilates renal and mesenteric vessels • Little direct cardiac action at this dose range 5-10 mcg/kg/min: • Predominant beta-adrenergic stimulating properties → increased force of contraction → increased cardiac output 10-20 mcg/kg/min: • Alpha effects dominate → renal, mesenteric, peripheral arterial and venous constriction → increased systemic vascular resistance and preload, increased heart rate	Hypotension and poor perfusion following resuscitation Shock unresponsive to fluid administration	Administered by IV infusion, never as a bolus 2-20 mcg/kg/min, titrated to desired effect. 10 ml/hr or 10 mcg/kg/min is a reasonable starting dose for the child with shock. Epinephrine is preferable to a dopamine infusion of more than 20 mcg/kg/min[6] To prepare infusion: 6 x body weight in kilograms = # of mg of dopamine to be added to a solution for a total volume of 100 ml (6 x kg = mg) Then: 1 ml/hr = 1 mcg/kg/min 2 ml/hr = 2 mcg/kg/min	• May induce tachycardia, ventricular ectopy and vasoconstriction. • Extravasation may result in tissue sloughing or necrosis - monitor IV site closely. • Inactivated by alkaline solutions. • Do not discontinue abruptly - taper gradually. • Administer via an infusion pump. • May not produce inotropic effects in catecholamine-depleted patients (chronic CHF, shock).

DRUG	MECHANISM OF ACTION/EFFECTS	INDICATIONS	DOSAGE	PRECAUTIONS
Dobutamine **Trade Name** Dobutrex **Class** Sympathomimetic Synthetic Catecholamine	Relatively selective beta-adrenergic stimulator • Potent inotropic effect (increased myocardial contractility → increased stroke volume → increased cardiac output) • Less chronotropic effect (heart rate) • Stimulates beta-2 receptors → peripheral vasodilation → decreased systemic vascular resistance	Low cardiac output and poor myocardial function following resuscitation	2-20 mcg/kg/min Patient response varies widely - monitor closely To prepare infusion: 6 x body weight in kilograms = # of mg of dobutamine to be added to a solution for a total volume of 100 ml (6 x kg = mg) Then: 1 ml/hr = 1 mcg/kg/min 2 ml/hr = 2 mcg/kg/min	May produce tachycardia, nausea, vomiting or ventricular ectopy. Do not mix with sodium bicarbonate - inactivates dobutamine. Do not discontinue abruptly - taper gradually. Administer via an infusion pump. Avoid in hypotensive patients. Vasodilatory effects may produce hypotension or fail to raise a low blood pressure.[7]

REFERENCES

1. Chameides, L., Hazinski MF (ed.), *Textbook of Pediatric Advanced Life Support.* Dallas: American Heart Association, 1994, p. 6-2.

2. Quan L., Seidel JS (ed.), *Instructor's Manual for Pediatric Advanced Life Support.* Dallas: American Heart Association, 1994, p. 4-13.

3. Chameides, L., Hazinski MF (ed.), *Textbook of Pediatric Advanced Life Support.* Dallas: American Heart Association, 1994, p. 7-5.

4. Chameides, L., Hazinski MF (ed.), *Textbook of Pediatric Advanced Life Support.* Dallas: American Heart Association, 1994, p. 6-8.

5. Chameides, L., Hazinski MF (ed.), *Textbook of Pediatric Advanced Life Support.* Dallas: American Heart Association, 1994, p. 6-13.

6. Chameides, L., Hazinski MF (ed.), *Textbook of Pediatric Advanced Life Support.* Dallas: American Heart Association, 1994, p. 6-13.

7. Quan L., Seidel JS (ed.), *Instructor's Manual for Pediatric Advanced Life Support.* Dallas: American Heart Association, 1994, p. 4-15.

Rhythm Disturbances 6

BASIC ELECTROPHYSIOLOGY

Definitions	1. Dysrhythmia = abnormal rhythm
	2. Arrhythmia = absence of rhythm
	Terms are used interchangeably
Myocardial Cell Types	1. Myocardial (working) cells (mechanical cells)
	• Contain contractile filaments that contract when the cells are electrically stimulated
	2. Electrical cells (pacemaker cells)
	• Electrical conduction system cells form and conduct impulses very rapidly

Action Potential	Electrical impulses are the result of brief but rapid flow of positively charged ions (primarily sodium) back and forth across the cell membrane

DOMINANT AND ESCAPE PACEMAKERS OF THE HEART

Primary Pacemaker	1. Normally the pacemaker cells with the fastest rate control the heart at any given time
	2. The SA (sino-atrial) node is normally the primary pacemaker of the heart because it possesses the highest level of automaticity
Escape Pacemakers	1. Atrio-Ventricular (AV) Junction
	If the SA node fails to generate an impulse at its normal rate, or stops functioning entirely, pacemaker cells in the AV junction will usually assume the role of pacemaker of the heart (but at a slower rate)
	2. Ventricles
	If the AV junction is unable to function, an escape pacemaker below the AV junction (the bundle branches and Purkinje network) may take over at an even slower rate

THE ELECTROCARDIOGRAM

P Wave	Represents atrial depolarization
PR Interval	The PR interval represents the length of time required for the atria to depolarize and the delay of the impulse through the AV junction
QRS Complex	Represents ventricular depolarization
	1. The Q wave is the first **negative** deflection following the P wave
	2. The R wave is the first **positive** deflection following the P wave
	3. The S wave is the **negative** deflection following the R wave
ST Segment	The ST segment begins with the end of the QRS complex and ends with onset of the T wave
T wave	Represents ventricular repolarization
QT Interval	Represents total ventricular activity (the time required for ventricular depolarization and repolarization to take place)

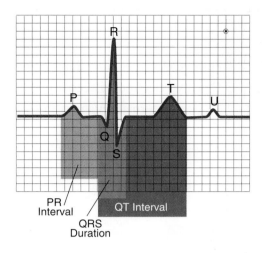

Figure 6-1. The electrocardiogram.

ABSOLUTE AND RELATIVE REFRACTORY PERIODS

Definition	The time between the onset of depolarization and the end of repolarization results in periods during which cardiac cells may or may not be stimulated to depolarize. These are known as the absolute and relative refractory periods.
Absolute Refractory Period	1. Extends from the onset of the QRS to the peak of the T wave
	2. Cardiac cells have not yet repolarized and cannot be stimulated to depolarize
	3. Also known as the effective refractory period
Relative Refractory Period	1. Corresponds with the downslope of the T wave
	2. Most of the cardiac cells have repolarized and can be stimulated to depolarize if the stimulus is strong enough
	3. Also known as the vulnerable period

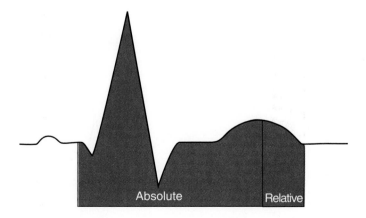

Figure 6-2. The absolute and relative refractory periods.

LEAD SYSTEMS

Lead I

- Positive electrode placed just below the left clavicle
- Negative electrode placed just below the right clavicle
- Provides information about the left lateral wall of the heart

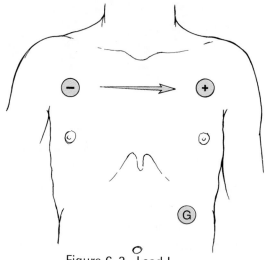

Figure 6-3. Lead I.

Lead II

- Positive electrode just below the left pectoral muscle
- Negative electrode just below the right clavicle
- Provides information about the inferior wall of the heart

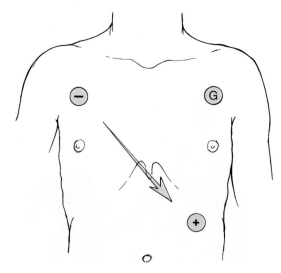

Figure 6-4. Lead II.

Lead III

- Positive electrode placed just below the left pectoral muscle
- Negative electrode placed just below the left clavicle
- Provides information about the inferior wall of the heart
- P waves seen in this lead are usually of lower amplitude than in Leads I and II and are more likely to be biphasic (partly positive and partly negative)

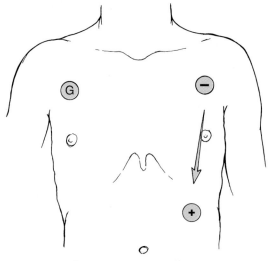

Figure 6-5. Lead III.

ANALYZING A RHYTHM STRIP

Determining Heart Rate

1. Is the rate fast, slow or within normal limits for the child's age?
   a. Tachycardia = faster than the upper range of normal for age
   b. Bradycardia = slower than the lower range of normal for age
2. For more precise determination of heart rate:
   a. Count the number of complete R waves within a period of 6 seconds and multiply that number by 10 to find the rate for one minute.
   b. Count the number of large squares (5 small boxes) between two R waves and divide into 300. This method is best used if the rhythm is regular, however, it may be used if the rhythm is irregular and a rate range (slowest and fastest rate) is given.
3. Pediatric patients can have extremely rapid heart rates that are difficult to count. When caring for an infant or child, a cardiac monitor that provides a continuous display of the child's heart rate is beneficial.

Is the rhythm regular or irregular?	1. If the rhythm is regular, the intervals between R waves will measure the same.
	2. If the atrial rhythm is regular, the intervals between P waves will measure the same.
Is the QRS wide or narrow?	1. The duration of the QRS is short in the infant and increases with age.
	2. If the QRS measures 0.08 second or less (narrow), it is presumed to be supraventricular in origin.
	3. If the QRS is greater than 0.08 second (wide), it is presumed to be ventricular in origin until proven otherwise.

Table 6-1. QRS Duration: Average and Upper Limits for Age.[1]

Age	Average QRS Duration	Upper Limit
0-1 month	0.05 sec	0.07 sec
1-6 months	0.05 sec	0.07 sec
6 mo-1 year	0.05 sec	0.07 sec
1-3 years	0.06 sec	0.07 sec
3-8 years	0.07 sec	0.08 sec
8-12 years	0.07 sec	0.09 sec
12-16 years	0.07 sec	0.10 sec
Adult	0.08 sec	0.10 sec

RHYTHM RECOGNITION

TACHYDYSRHYTHMIAS

Sinus Tachycardia	Rate:	Faster than upper limit of normal for age, usually less than 200 beats/minute
	Rhythm:	Usually regular but may vary
	P waves:	Upright in Lead II, if discernible
	QRS:	Within normal limits (narrow)
	Cause:	Anxiety, fear, fever, hypovolemia, pain, catecholamines, hypoxemia
	Significance:	Increased myocardial workload usually well tolerated by the healthy heart. Chest x-ray usually normal, depending on the cause of the tachycardia.
	Treatment:	Identify and treat the underlying cause

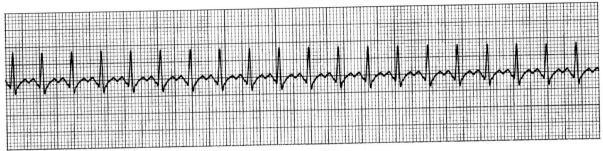

Figure 6-6. Sinus Tachycardia.

Supraventricular
Tachycardia (SVT)

Rate: 240 ±40 beats/minute[2]; may be as high as 300 beats/minute in infants

Rhythm: Regular

P waves: Often indiscernible due to rapid rate; may be lost in the T wave of the preceding beat

QRS: Within normal limits (less than 0.08 sec)

Cause: Most often due to reentrant mechanism

Significance: 1. Cardiac output = heart rate x stroke volume. Tachydysrhythmias result in low cardiac output due to a fast heart rate and low stroke volume as a result of decreased ventricular filling time.

2. Most common tachydysrhythmia seen in the pediatric patient. Onset and termination of the rhythm are often abrupt (paroxysmal).

Treatment: Adenosine, synchronized countershock depending on stability of the patient.

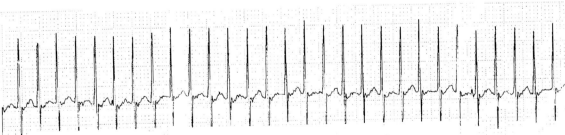

Figure 6-7. Supraventricular tachycardia.

Ventricular Tachycardia (VT)	Rate:	120-400 beats/minute
	Rhythm:	Essentially regular
	P waves:	Usually not seen; if present, they have no set relationship to the QRS's appearing between the QRS complexes at a rate different from that of the VT
	QRS:	> 0.08 sec (wide); may be difficult to differentiate between the QRS and the T wave
	T waves:	Usually opposite in polarity to the QRS
	Cause:	May be caused by hypoxia, acidosis, electrolyte imbalance, reactions to medications or ingestion of poisons (such as cyclic antidepressants)
	Significance:	1. Uncommon dysrhythmia in the pediatric patient.
		2. Slow rates may be well tolerated but rapid rates often result in decreased ventricular filling time, decreasing cardiac output, possibly degenerating into ventricular fibrillation.
	Treatment:	Lidocaine, synchronized countershock depending on stability of the patient. Defibrillation if pulseless.

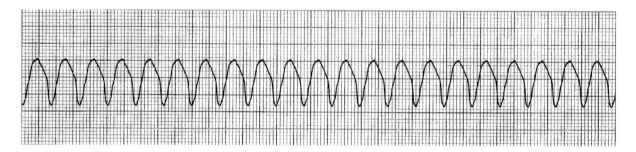

Figure 6-8. Ventricular tachycardia.

Table 6-2. Differentiation of Sinus Tachycardia and Supraventricular Tachycardia.		
Rate	Sinus Tachycardia < 200 (variable rate)	Supraventricular Tachycardia > 220 (constant rate)
History	Fever, volume loss due to trauma, vomiting, diarrhea, pain	Usually abrupt onset with nonspecific signs - irritability, lethargy, poor feeding
Physical Examination	May be consistent with volume loss Possible fever Clear lungs Normal-sized liver	Signs of poor perfusion including diminished peripheral pulses, delayed capillary refill, pallor, tachypnea, possible crackles, enlarged liver

Differentiation of Wide-QRS SVT and Ventricular Tachycardia

1. Wide-QRS SVT is relatively uncommon in infants and children.
2. Any wide-QRS tachycardia should be presumed to be ventricular in origin and treated as ventricular tachycardia.

BRADYDYSRHYTHMIAS

Bradycardias

Rate: Slower than the lower range of normal for age

Rhythm: Usually regular

P waves: May or may not be present; relationship between the P wave and QRS complexes may be lost

QRS: May be narrow or wide depending on the site of origin of the bradycardia

Cause: Hypoxia, acidosis, hypotension, increased vagal tone (suctioning)

Significance: 1. Cardiac output = heart rate x stroke volume. Bradydysrhythmias result in low cardiac output due to a low heart rate, despite normal stroke volume. May degenerate to cardiac arrest.

2. Most common preterminal rhythms in the pediatric patient:
   - Sinus bradycardia
   - Sinus arrest with a slow junctional or ventricular escape rhythm
   - Various degrees of AV block

3. Note: Bradycardia (heart rate less than 60 beats/minute) with poor systemic perfusion should be treated in a child of any age, even if blood pressure is normal.[3]

Treatment: Ensure good oxygenation and ventilation. Begin chest compressions if heart rate <60/min in an infant or child with poor systemic perfusion despite oxygenation and ventilation. Establish IV or IO access. Epinephrine, atropine, possible transcutaneous pacing.

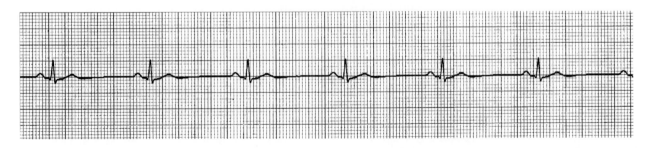

Figure 6-9. Sinus bradycardia.

ABSENT COLLAPSE, DISORGANIZED RHYTHMS

Asystole (Ventricular Asystole, Ventricular Standstill)

Rate: Ventricular usually not discernible but may see some atrial activity

Rhythm: Atrial may be discernible, ventricular not discernible

P waves: Usually not discernible

QRS: Absent

Significance: Absence of cardiac output. Patient unconscious, pulseless and apneic.

Treatment: Confirm the patient is pulseless and apneic. Confirm the rhythm in another lead. Begin CPR and ACLS management.

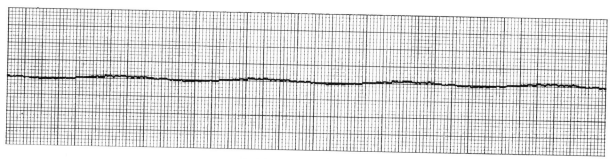

Figure 6-10. Asystole.

Ventricular Fibrillation (VF)

Rate: Cannot be determined since there are no discernible waves or complexes to measure

Rhythm: Rapid and chaotic with no pattern or regularity

P waves: Not discernible

QRS: Not discernible

Cause: Severe hypoxia and/or poor perfusion, electrolyte imbalance, hypothermia, drug toxicity (digitalis, cyclic antidepressants)

Significance: Terminal rhythm. Uncommon in children and even more rare in infants. Patient unconscious, pulseless and apneic.

Treatment: Confirm the patient is pulseless and apneic. Check leads. Initiate ventilation, oxygenation and chest compressions until a defibrillator is available.

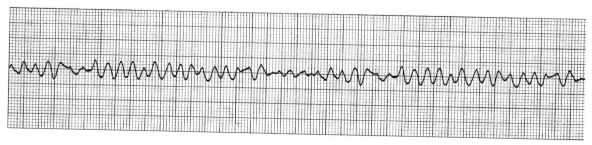

Figure 6-11. Ventricular fibrillation.

Pulseless Electrical Activity (PEA) formerly known as Electromechanical Dissociation (EMD)

1. Definition: organized electrical activity without palpable pulses
2. Causes: PATH(x3)
   - Pneumothorax (tension), Acidosis, Tamponade (cardiac), Hypoxemia (severe), Hypovolemia (severe), Hypothermia (profound)
3. Treatment: Confirm the patient is pulseless and apneic. Begin BLS and ACLS management. Look for underlying cause and correct if present.

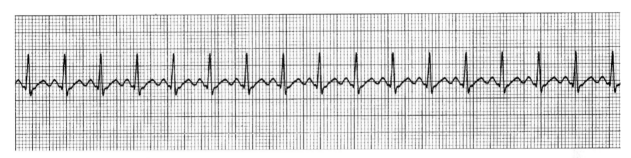

Figure 6-12. Pulseless electrical activity - organized electrical activity without a palpable pulse.

ELECTRICAL THERAPY

Terminology

Countershock and cardioversion are GENERAL terms. Verbalize specifically what TYPE of shock will be delivered:
- Unsynchronized countershock = defibrillation
  - The delivery of energy has no relationship to the cardiac cycle
- Synchronized countershock
  - The delivery of energy is timed within milliseconds of the R wave in the cardiac cycle

FACTORS AFFECTING TRANSTHORACIC RESISTANCE (IMPEDANCE)

Delivered Energy

The higher the energy used for countershock, the lower the transthoracic resistance.

Paddle Size

To a point, transthoracic resistance decreases with increased paddle size. Recommended paddle sizes:[4]
- 4.5 cm paddles (infant paddles) should be used for infants up to approximately 1 year of age or 10 kg
- 8-13 cm paddles (adult paddles) should be used for patients older than 1 year or weighing more than 10 kg.

Paddle-Skin Interface

1. The skin acts as an electrical resistor between the paddles and the heart.
2. If interface is not used:
   - Skin surface burns
   - Lack of penetration of current
3. Types of interface most frequently used include electrode cream or paste, disposable defib pads or self-adhesive monitoring-defibrillation pads.

Number and Interval between Previous Shocks

1. The effect of the number of countershocks delivered on transthoracic resistance is cumulative.
2. Transthoracic resistance is also affected by the interval between successive shocks.
   - In pulseless VT or VF, three "stacked" shocks are delivered

Paddle Pressure

1. Firm paddle pressure may further decrease transthoracic resistance.
2. Exertion of firm pressure on the paddles may act to decrease transthoracic resistance by forcing exhalation.

Phase of Patient's Ventilation

1. Air is a poor conductor of electricity.
2. Transthoracic resistance may be lowest when countershock is performed during the expiratory phase of respiration because the distance between the paddles and the heart is decreased.

Paddle Distance

1. The recommended position for paddle placement is placement of one paddle on the upper right chest below the clavicle and the other just to the left of the left nipple in the anterior axillary line (over the apex of the heart).

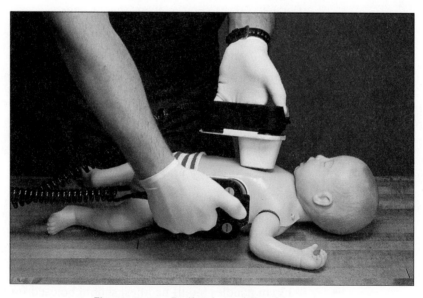

Figure 6-13. Pediatric paddle placement.

2. Anterior-posterior paddle positioning may also be used. One paddle is placed on the anterior chest over the heart and the other is positioned behind the heart.

If pediatric paddles are unavailable and adult paddles are used, the anterior-posterior paddle position should be used.

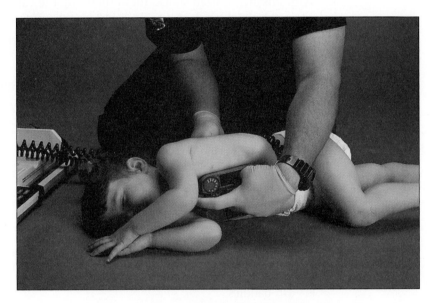

Figure 6-14. Anterior-posterior paddle positioning.

QUICK-LOOK

Procedure

1. Apply gel to defibrillator paddles or defibrillator pads to the patient's chest
2. Turn the lead selector on the monitor/defibrillator to "paddles"
3. Apply the paddles to the patient's chest
   - The paddles will function as electrodes, monitoring the patient's cardiac rhythm
   - Caution: removal of the paddles from the patient's chest while in "paddle" mode will result in artifact display on the cardiac monitor. The paddles must remain in contact with the patient's chest to monitor the patient's cardiac rhythm.

DEFIBRILLATION

Purpose

1. Defibrillation does not "jump start" the heart
2. The purpose of defibrillation is to produce momentary asystole
   - The shock attempts to completely depolarize the myocardium and provide an opportunity for the natural pacemaker centers of the heart to resume normal activity
3. With unsynchronized shocks (defibrillation), the capacitors discharge when the shock controls (discharge buttons) are depressed
   - Unsynchronized shocks have no relationship to the cardiac cycle
4. Electric shocks produce parasympathetic discharge
   - Routine shocking of asystole is strongly discouraged
   - Shocking asystole could eliminate any possibility for return of spontaneous cardiac activity

Indications

1. Ventricular fibrillation
2. Pulseless ventricular tachycardia

Operating the Defibrillator

1. Locate on/off switches
2. Patient leads
3. Quick-look (paddles used as electrodes)
4. Select appropriate energy level for patient weight
5. Locate charge button
   - On paddles
   - On machine
6. Locate discharge buttons
7. Hands-free defibrillation

Procedure

1. Apply conductive material to the paddles (gel) or chest wall (defib pads)
   - Alcohol pads should not be used because they are a fire hazard and may cause serious burns
2. Turn on the defibrillator
3. Select appropriate energy level for patient weight
4. Place paddles on the chest and apply firm pressure
5. Charge paddles
6. State and LOOK to be sure area is clear
   a. Look all around (360-degrees)
   b. Call "all clear!"
7. Press both discharge buttons simultaneously to deliver shock
8. Evaluate ECG.

SYNCHRONIZED COUNTERSHOCK (CARDIOVERSION)

Purpose

1. Synchronized countershock reduces the potential for delivery of energy during the vulnerable period of the T wave (relative refractory period)
2. A synchronizing circuit allows the delivery of a countershock to be "programmed"
   a. Searches for the peak of the QRS complex (R wave deflection)
   b. Delivers the shock a few milliseconds after the highest part of the R wave

Indications

1. Unstable supraventricular tachycardia (SVT)
2. Unstable ventricular tachycardia (VT) with a pulse

Procedure

1. Apply conductive material to the paddles (gel) or chest wall (defib pads)
   - Alcohol pads should not be used because they are a fire hazard and may cause serious burns
2. Turn on the defibrillator
3. Select appropriate energy level for patient weight
4. Press synchronizer switch/button
5. Assure machine sensing of the R wave
6. Place paddles on the chest and apply firm pressure
7. Charge paddles
8. State and LOOK to be sure area is clear
   a. Look all around (360-degrees)
   b. Call "all clear!"
9. Press both discharge buttons simultaneously to deliver shock

NONINVASIVE (TRANSCUTANEOUS) PACING

Indications   Class IIb (possibly helpful) for the child with profound symptomatic bradycardia refractory to basic and advanced life support therapy.

Description   Equipment requirements for performing the procedure include an external pacemaker and two large adhesive-backed electrodes.

1. Pediatric electrodes (small or medium) should be used if the child weighs less than 15 kg.

2. The negative electrode is placed on the anterior chest over the heart. The positive electrode is placed on the back behind the heart.

    a. If the back cannot be used, the positive electrode should be placed on the anterior chest under the right clavicle and the negative electrode on the left side of the chest over the fourth intercostal space in the midaxillary line.

    b. "Precise placement of electrodes does not appear to be necessary provided that the negative electrode is placed near the apex of the heart."[5]

PATIENT MANAGEMENT

BRADYCARDIAS

Assess ABCs
Secure the airway
Administer 100% oxygen
Assess vital signs
↓
Severe cardiorespiratory compromise?
Poor perfusion
Hypotension
Respiratory difficulty

NO
↓
Patient observation
Support ABCs
Consider transfer or transport to ALS facility

YES
↓
Perform chest compressions if, despite oxygenation and ventilation:
Heart rate is <60/min in infant or
child associated with poor systemic perfusion

(Special considerations may apply in the presence of severe hypothermia)
↓

Establish IV or intraosseous (IO) access
↓

Epinephrine
IV/IO: 0.01 mg/kg of 1:10,000 solution (0.1 ml/kg)
ET: 0.1 mg/kg of 1:1000 solution (0.1 ml/kg)
Repeat every 3-5 minutes at same dose
↓

Atropine
0.02 mg/kg
Minimum dose 0.1 mg
Maximum single dose: 0.5 mg for child, 1.0 mg for adolescent
(may be repeated once)
↓

Consider transcutaneous pacing

TACHYDYSRHYTHMIAS

Sinus Tachycardia

Assess ABCs
Ensure effective oxygenation and ventilation
Treat underlying cause

Supraventricular
Tachycardia
- Stable Patient

Assess ABCs
Secure the airway
Administer oxygen
Establish intravenous access
Initiate continuous ECG monitoring
Administer adenosine 0.1 mg/kg rapid IV bolus
If no effect, the initial dose may be doubled
Maximum single dose of adenosine is 12 mg

Ventricular Tachycardia
- Stable Patient

Assess ABCs
Secure the airway
Administer oxygen
Establish intravenous access
Initiate continuous ECG monitoring
Administer lidocaine 1 mg/kg IV bolus over 1-2 minutes

Supraventricular
Tachycardia or Ventricular
Tachycardia -
Unstable Patient

Unstable:
• Congestive heart failure
• Diminished peripheral
  perfusion
• Hypotension

Assess ABCs
Secure the airway
Administer 100% oxygen
Establish IV or intraosseous (IO) access
Assess vital signs
Initiate continuous ECG monitoring
Correct hypoxemia, acidosis, hypoglycemia or hypothermia if present
Perform synchronized countershock with 0.5 joules/kg
Check pulse and reassess rhythm
If unsuccessful, perform synchronized countershock with 1 joule/kg
Check pulse and reassess rhythm

Adenosine may be administered before synchronized countershock in unstable SVT if IV access is readily available, however, cardioversion should not be delayed to obtain IV access.

If readily available, lidocaine should be administered for ventricular tachycardia before synchronized countershock, however, defibrillation should not be delayed if IV access or lidocaine is not readily available.

ABSENT (COLLAPSE OR DISORGANIZED) RHYTHMS

Ventricular Fibrillation or
Pulseless Ventricular Tachycardia

Search for:
- Metabolic abnormality (calcium, potassium, magnesium or glucose imbalance)
- Hypothermia
- Drug toxicity (digitalis, cyclic antidepressants)

Determine pulselessness and begin CPR
Confirm cardiac rhythm in more than one lead
↓
Continue CPR
Secure the airway
Hyperventilate with 100% oxygen
Establish IV or intraosseous (IO) access but do not delay defibrillation
↓
Defibrillate up to 3 times if needed
2 joules/kg
4 joules/kg
4 joules/kg
↓
Epinephrine (initial dose)
IV/IO: 0.01 mg/kg of 1:10,000 solution (0.1 ml/kg)
ET: 0.1 mg/kg of 1:1000 solution (0.1 ml/kg)
↓
Defibrillate with 4 j/kg within 30-60 seconds
↓
Lidocaine
1 mg/kg IV or IO
↓
Defibrillate with 4 j/kg within 30-60 seconds
↓
Epinephrine (second and subsequent doses)
IV/IO/ET: 0.1 mg/kg of 1:1000 solution (0.1 ml/kg)
Repeat every 3-5 minutes
(IV/IO doses of up to 0.2 mg/kg of 1:1000 solution may be effective)
↓
Defibrillate with 4 j/kg within 30-60 seconds
↓
Lidocaine
1 mg/kg IV or IO
↓
Defibrillate with 4 j/kg within 30-60 seconds
↓
Consider **Bretylium**
5 mg/kg IV first dose
10 mg/kg IV second dose

Defibrillate with 4 j/kg after EACH medication

Asystole

Determine pulselessness and begin CPR
Confirm cardiac rhythm in more than one lead
↓
Continue CPR
Secure the airway
Hyperventilate with 100% oxygen
Establish IV or intraosseous (IO) access
↓
Epinephrine (initial dose)
IV/IO: 0.01 mg/kg of 1:10,000 solution (0.1 ml/kg)
ET: 0.1 mg/kg of 1:1000 solution (0.1 ml/kg)
↓
Epinephrine (second and subsequent doses)
IV/IO/ET: 0.1 mg/kg of 1:1000 solution (0.1 ml/kg)
Repeat every 3-5 minutes
(IV/IO doses of up to 0.2 mg/kg of 1:1000 solution may be effective)

Pulseless Electrical Activity (PEA)

Determine pulselessness and begin CPR
Confirm cardiac rhythm in more than one lead
↓
Rule out treatable causes: PATH(x3)
Pneumothorax (tension)
Acidosis (severe)
Tamponade (cardiac)
Hypoxemia (severe)
Hypovolemia (severe)
Hypothermia (profound)
↓
Continue CPR
Secure the airway
Hyperventilate with 100% oxygen
Establish IV or intraosseous (IO) access
↓
Epinephrine (initial dose)
IV/IO: 0.01 mg/kg of 1:10,000 solution (0.1 ml/kg)
ET: 0.1 mg/kg of 1:1000 solution (0.1 ml/kg)
↓
Epinephrine (second and subsequent doses)
IV/IO/ET: 0.1 mg/kg of 1:1000 solution (0.1 ml/kg)
Repeat every 3-5 minutes
(IV/IO doses of up to 0.2 mg/kg of 1:1000 solution may be effective)

REFERENCES

1. Park, M. *The Pediatric Cardiology Handbook.* St. Louis: Mosby-Year Book, 1991.

2. Park, M. *The Pediatric Cardiology Handbook.* St. Louis: Mosby-Year Book, 1991.

3. Chameides, L., Hazinski MF (ed.), *Textbook of Pediatric Advanced Life Support.* Dallas: American Heart Association, 1994, p. 7-6.

4. Chameides, L., Hazinski MF (ed.), *Textbook of Pediatric Advanced Life Support.* Dallas: American Heart Association, 1994, p. 7-10.

5. Chameides, L., Hazinski MF (ed.), *Textbook of Pediatric Advanced Life Support.* Dallas: American Heart Association, 1994, p. 7-11.

QUIZ – FLUIDS, MEDICATIONS AND RHYTHM DISTURBANCES

1. Synchronized countershock:

    a. is used only for unstable supraventricular tachycardia
    b. delivers a shock between the peak and end of the T wave
    c. is timed to avoid the vulnerable period of the cardiac cycle
    d. is used only for rhythms with a ventricular response < 100/minute

2. Drowsiness, disorientation, muscle twitching and seizures are adverse effects that may result from administration of:

    a. atropine
    b. lidocaine
    c. bretylium
    d. adenosine

3. In which of the following situations is unsynchronized countershock suggested?

    1. asystole
    2. symptomatic bradycardia
    3. pulseless ventricular tachycardia
    4. pulseless electrical activity
    5. ventricular fibrillation

    a. 1, 2
    b. 3, 5
    c. 1, 3, 4
    d. 2, 4, 5

4. The primary pacemaker of the heart is normally the:

    a. SA node
    b. ventricles
    c. AV junction
    d. bundle of His

5. The initial fluid bolus for restoration of blood volume should be:

    a. 10 ml/kg of crystalloid solution
    b. 20 ml/kg of crystalloid solution
    c. 10 ml/kg of 5% dextrose in water
    d. 20 ml/kg of 5% dextrose in water

6.　Atropine sulfate:

    a.　is the drug of choice for supraventricular tachycardia

    b.　decreases heart rate (slows sinus or atrial pacemakers) and AV conduction

    c.　is considered a Class I (definitely helpful) intervention in symptomatic bradycardia with AV block (uncommon event) and vagally mediated bradycardia during intubation attempts

    d.　is considered a Class IIb (possibly helpful) intervention after defibrillation, epinephrine and lidocaine have failed to convert ventricular fibrillation or pulseless ventricular tachycardia

Questions 7-10 refer to the following scenario.

    A pulseless and apneic six year old male is brought by ambulance to your Emergency Department. Basic EMTs report the child was the front-seat passenger of a vehicle involved in a rollover accident. The child was not restrained. Examination confirms the child to be pulseless and apneic with contusions noted on the anterior chest and open fractures of both femurs. Chest compressions are being performed and the patient is being ventilated with 100% oxygen via a bag-valve device. The cardiac monitor displays the following rhythm:

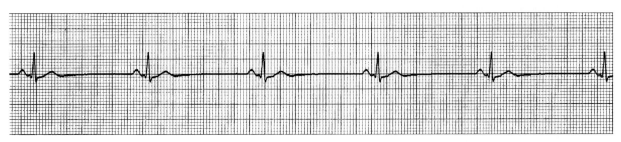

Figure 6-15.

7.　The rhythm displayed above is _____.

8.　The patient is unconscious, pulseless and apneic. This clinical situation is termed:

    a.　asystole

    b.　ventricular fibrillation

    c.　pulseless electrical activity

    d.　pulseless ventricular tachycardia

9.　List five (5) possible causes of the clinical situation presented above.

    1.　_____

    2.　_____

    3.　_____

    4.　_____

    5.　_____

10. A first-line medication suggested in this situation is:

    a. atropine
    b. dopamine
    c. epinephrine
    d. sodium bicarbonate

11. The recommended endotracheal dose of epinephrine is:

    a. 0.1 mg/kg of 1:1000 solution
    b. 0.2 mg/kg of 1:1000 solution
    c. 0.01 mg/kg of 1:10,000 solution
    d. 0.02 mg/kg of 1:10,000 solution

12. Select the **INCORRECT** statement regarding the management of symptomatic bradycardia.

    a. hypoxia is a common cause of bradycardia in the pediatric patient
    b. it is important to administer a vagolytic dose of atropine because smaller doses may produce paradoxical tachycardia
    c. atropine should be used to treat bradycardia only after adequate oxygenation and ventilation have been assured
    d. bradycardia (heart rate less than 80 beats per minute) associated with poor systemic perfusion should be treated in a child of any age, even if blood pressure is normal

13. Increased heart rate and force of myocardial contraction are effects that occur with stimulation of:

    a. beta-1 receptors
    b. beta-2 receptors
    c. alpha-1 receptors
    d. dopaminergic receptors

14. Bretylium tosylate is used in the management of:

    a. sinus tachycardia
    b. symptomatic bradycardia
    c. VF refractory to lidocaine
    d. supraventricular tachycardia

15. Adenosine:

    a. is a first-line agent in the management of supraventricular tachycardia
    b. increases systolic blood pressure and dilates the renal and mesenteric vasculature
    c. is an electrolyte useful in the treatment of documented or suspected hypocalcemia
    d. is a pure beta-adrenergic stimulator that produces an increase in heart rate, conduction velocity and cardiac contractility

16. Wide-QRS tachycardias in an infant or child should be presumed to be:

    a. sinus tachycardia
    b. ventricular fibrillation
    c. ventricular tachycardia
    d. supraventricular tachycardia

17. Administration of glucose is considered a Class I (definitely helpful) intervention in:
    a. ventricular fibrillation
    b. symptomatic bradycardia
    c. documented cases of hypoglycemia
    d. shock associated with metabolic acidosis

18. The recommended continuous infusion rate for lidocaine is:
    a. 1-2 mg/min
    b. 2-20 mg/kg/min
    c. 20-50 mcg/kg/min
    d. 0.1-1.0 mcg/kg/min

19. Which of the following is an example of paddle-skin interface that should NOT be used?
    a. alcohol pads
    b. electrode cream or paste
    c. disposable defibrillation pads
    d. self-adhesive monitoring-defibrillation pads

20. Pediatric rhythm disturbances may be categorized as fast, slow or absent (collapse) rhythms. List three examples of rhythm disturbances found in the absent rhythm category.

    1. _____

    2. _____

    3. _____

QUIZ ANSWERS – FLUIDS, MEDICATIONS AND RHYTHM DISTURBANCES

QUESTION	ANSWER	RATIONALE	STUDY GUIDE REFERENCE	PALS PAGE REFERENCE
1	C	Synchronized countershock delivers a shock a few milliseconds after the highest part of the R wave, thus avoiding the vulnerable period of the cardiac cycle. Delivery of synchronized countershock is suggested for the unstable patient in supraventricular or ventricular tachycardia (with a pulse).	165	7-4
2	B	Excessive doses of lidocaine may produce myocardial and circulatory depression and central nervous system symptoms including drowsiness, dizziness, disorientation and focal or generalized seizures.	147	6-14
3	B	Unsynchronized countershock (defibrillation) is indicated for ventricular fibrillation and pulseless ventricular tachycardia. Defibrillation has not been shown to be effective in the treatment of asystole.	164	7-8
4	A	The primary pacemaker of the heart is normally the SA (sino-atrial) node.	152	7-1
5	B	20 ml/kg of crystalloid solution should be administered when vascular access is obtained to restore blood volume. This amount should be administered as a bolus in less than 20 minutes.	140	6-2

6	C	Atropine is considered a Class I (definitely helpful) intervention in symptomatic bradycardia with AV block (uncommon event) and vagally mediated bradycardia during intubation attempts. Atropine **increases** heart rate (accelerates sinus or atrial pacemakers) and improves AV conduction. Atropine is not indicated in the management of VF or pulseless VT. **Adenosine** is the drug of choice for SVT.	146	6-6
7		The rhythm shown is a sinus bradycardia.	159	N/A
8	C	Despite the presence of a rhythm on the cardiac monitor, the patient is pulseless. This situation is termed pulseless electrical activity (electro-mechanical dissociation).	161	7-9
9		Possible causes of pulseless electrical activity include: PATH(x3) Pneumothorax (tension) Acidosis (severe) Tamponade (cardiac) Hypoxemia (severe) Hypovolemia (severe) Hypothermia (profound)	161, 170	7-9
10	C	Epinephrine is a first-line medication indicated in the management of pulseless electrical activity.	143, 170	7-9
11	A	The recommended endotracheal dose of epinephrine 0.1 mg/kg of 1:1000 solution - 10 times the IV/IO dose.	143	6-6
12	B	It is important to administer a vagolytic dose of atropine because smaller doses may produce paradoxical bradycardia. The recommended dose of atropine is 0.02 mg/kg with a minimum dose of 0.1 mg.	146	6-8

13	A	Increased heart rate and force of myocardial contraction are effects that occur with stimulation of beta-1 adrenergic receptors.	138	N/A
14	C	Bretylium tosylate (Bretylol) is a ventricular antidysrhythmic used in the management of ventricular fibrillation refractory to defibrillation and lidocaine.	147	7-6
15	A	Adenosine (Adenocard) is an endogenous chemical that causes a temporary block through the AV node and interrupts reentry circuits that involve the AV node and that are responsible for the vast majority of SVT episodes in infants and children.	145	7-5
16	C	Wide-QRS tachycardia in an infant or child should be presumed to be ventricular tachycardia until proven otherwise.	156, 159	7-5
17	C	Glucose (dextrose) is considered a Class I (definitely helpful) intervention in cases of documented hypoglycemia.	144	6-10
18	C	The recommended continuous infusion rate for lidocaine is 20-50 mcg/kg/minute. A bolus of lidocaine should be administered before initiation of a continuous infusion to assure adequate plasma concentrations.	147	6-14
19	A	Alcohol pads should not be used as they are a fire hazard and may cause serious chest burns.	164, 165	7-10
20		Examples of absent (disorganized or collapse) rhythms include ventricular fibrillation or pulseless ventricular tachycardia, asystole and pulseless electrical activity.	160-161, 169-170	7-6

BREATHING

100% Inspired Oxygen

Administer 100% oxygen unless hyperoxygenation is reflected by direct PaO_2 measurement

Children who remain agitated despite effective mechanical ventilation may require sedation (midazolam or diazepam), analgesia or paralytics (vecuronium or pancuronium) with analgesia (morphine or fentanyl) to:

- Optimize ventilation
- Reduce risk of barotrauma
- Reduce risk of accidental endotracheal tube dislodgment

Mechanical Ventilation

Obtain arterial blood gas after 10-15 minutes on initial ventilator settings. Adjust accordingly.

1. Initial rate of mechanical or manual ventilation should be:
   a. 20-30 breaths/minute for infants (normal lungs)
   b. 16-20 breaths/minute for older children (normal lungs)
      - If intrinsic pulmonary disease or intracranial hypertension is present, higher rates may be needed
      - Lower respiratory rates should be used in those patients with asthma, bronchiolitis or other conditions involving air-trapping to provide adequate exhalation time

2. Initial tidal volume should be 10-15 ml/kg
   a. Assess adequacy of tidal volume by evaluation of chest expansion and bilateral breath sounds.
   b. Higher volumes will be needed if there is a significant air leak around the endotracheal tube.
      - May be necessary to replace the endotracheal tube with a larger one

3. Peak inspiratory pressure
   a. Begin at 20-30 cm H20 if lung compliance normal
   b. Increase slowly and gradually until chest expansion is observed and bilateral breath sounds are adequate.
      - Higher pressures may be required in the presence of lung disease.
   c. Inspiratory time should be 0.5-1.0 second

4. Positive end-expiratory pressure (PEEP)

    a. 2-4 cm H20 should be provided initially

    b. Higher levels may be needed if diffuse alveolar disease or marked ventilation-perfusion mismatch associated with hypoxemia is present.

Patient Assessment

1. Inspection

    a. Signs of increased work of breathing include:

        -   Tachypnea
        -   Head bobbing
        -   Nasal flaring
        -   Retractions
        -   Use of accessory muscles

    b. Agitation may reflect inadequate oxygenation or ventilation

    c. Cyanosis of mucous membranes is indicative of hypoxemia

2. Auscultation of breath sounds

    a. Should be equal bilaterally

    b. Unilateral breath sounds (especially on the right) may indicate right mainstem bronchus intubation but may also be due to:

        -   Mucous plug
        -   Pneumothorax
        -   Pleural effusion
        -   Lung consolidation
        -   Foreign body airway obstruction

    c. Pulmonary edema, infection, aspiration or bronchospasm may produce rales, rhonchi or wheezing.

Noninvasive Monitoring

1. All patients should be monitored by pulse oximetry

    -   CO_2 monitoring optional

2. Continued reevaluation of the patient is ESSENTIAL since these devices may be inaccurate in the presence of hypothermia or poor peripheral perfusion.

CARDIOVASCULAR SYSTEM

Circulation

After cessation of chest compressions, perform a rapid assessment of cardiovascular performance.

1. Persistent circulatory dysfunction is likely in the postresuscitation phase.

2. Cardiac output must be supported to assure adequate delivery of oxygen to the tissues.

3. Frequent assessment and initiation of appropriate therapy is necessary to prevent recurrent cardiopulmonary arrest.

Signs of Inadequate Systemic Perfusion	1. Decreased capillary refill
	2. Absence or decreased intensity of distal pulses
	3. Altered mental status
	4. Cool extremities
	5. Tachycardia
	6. Hypotension
	7. Decreased urine output
	a. Urine output is an indicator of renal perfusion
	b. May not be a reliable indicator if renal failure secondary to shock develops after resuscitation
Possible Causes of Decreased Cardiac Output	1. Insufficient volume resuscitation
	2. Loss of peripheral vascular tone (as seen in sepsis, anaphylaxis, neurogenic shock)
	3. Myocardial dysfunction with inadequate, or premature, withdrawal of support
	Treat with fluids or vasoactive agents
Patient Monitoring	1. Monitor heart rate, blood pressure and pulse oximetry
	• Assess at least every five minutes until stable, then every 15 minutes
	2. Cuff blood pressures may be inaccurate in the recently resuscitated child. Initiate direct arterial monitoring when possible in cases of continued cardiovascular compromise.
	• Normotension does not assure adequate cardiac output
	• Hypotension must be treated aggressively
	3. Urine output should be monitored with an indwelling catheter
Additional Studies	1. Arterial blood gases, serum electrolytes, calcium, glucose, serum urea nitrogen, creatinine, hematocrit
	• Metabolic acidosis suggests inadequate cardiac output
	2. Chest x-ray may help determine intravascular volume
	• Small heart consistent with hypovolemia
	• Large heart consistent with myocardial dysfunction or volume overload

CENTRAL NERVOUS SYSTEM

1. CNS dysfunction may be the cause or result of a cardiopulmonary arrest.

2. If signs of serious CNS depression are present, until intracranial pressure status can be comprehensively evaluated:
   - Intubate
   - Hyperventilate to maintain $PaCO_2$ at 22-29^2 mmHg

3. Adequate cerebral perfusion pressure is dependent upon maintenance of blood pressure and perfusion

4. Serial neurological assessments are essential

RENAL SYSTEM

Decreased urine output (< 1.0 ml/kg/hr or patients up to 30 kg) may result from:
- Prerenal causes
- Inadequate systemic perfusion
- Ischemic renal damage
  - Combination of these

1. Obtain baseline serum urea nitrogen and creatinine when possible.

2. Administer additional fluid if signs of volume depletion are present.

3. Treat myocardial dysfunction with catecholamine infusion.

4. Until renal status is determined, avoid or use caution when administering nephrotoxic and renally excreted medications.

GASTROINTESTINAL SYSTEM

1. Insert an orogastric or nasogastric tube to prevent or treat gastric distention if:
   a. Bowel sounds are absent
   b. Gastric distention is present
   c. Patient requires mechanical ventilation

2. Blind nasogastric tube placement is contraindicated in the patient with serious facial trauma.

GENERAL POSTRESUSCITATION CARE

Once the patient is stable:

1. Change intraosseous line to IV line(s).

2. Secure all IV lines.

3. Splint any fractures.

4. Treat the underlying cause of the arrest if known (infection, ingestion, etc.).

5. Monitor serum glucose and core body temperature frequently. Initiate appropriate measures as needed.

INTERHOSPITAL TRANSPORT

1. Postresuscitation care should be provided by trained medical personnel in pediatric intensive care units.

2. Transport team should be specifically trained and experienced in the care of critically ill and injured children.

3. Mode of transport and transport team members should be based on individual patient need.

4. The single most important factor in determining interhospital transport should be provision of the highest level of pediatric care during transport.

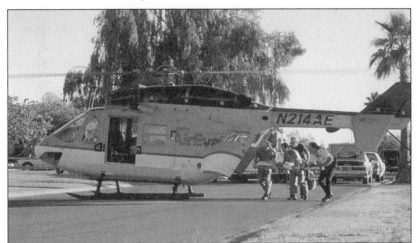

Figure 7-1 A and B.   The most important factor determining interhospital transport should be provision of the highest level of pediatric care during transport. (A from Sanders M., *Mosby's Paramedic Textbook*, St. Louis, 1994, Mosby–Year Book.) Photo by Colin Williams.

Neonatal Resuscitation 8

OBJECTIVES

Upon completion of this chapter, you will be able to:

1. Identify the primary phases of newborn resuscitation.
2. State antepartum and intrapartum factors associated with an increased risk for neonatal resuscitation.
3. Identify equipment items that should be readily available for resuscitation of a distressed newborn.
4. State methods by which heat loss may be prevented during newborn resuscitation.
5. Describe the possible consequences of prolonged suctioning attempts.
6. Describe safe methods for providing tactile stimulation to the neonate.
7. Name the objective signs used in determining an Apgar score.
8. State possible causes of a poor response to assisted ventilation efforts during resuscitation.
9. State the indications for performing endotracheal intubation in the newborn.
10. Describe signs of correct endotracheal tube placement.
11. Name complications that may occur for initiating chest compressions in the neonate.
12. State the heart rate conditions for initiating chest compressions in the neonate.
13. Describe the technique used for performing chest compressions in the neonate.
14. State the indications, mechanism of action, dosage and route of administration for epinephrine and naloxone.
15. Describe the indications for volume expanders in neonatal resuscitation.

Definition   Neonate = an infant less than 1 month of age

Phases of Newborn   1. Preparation
Resuscitation   2. Resuscitation
                               3. Postresuscitation

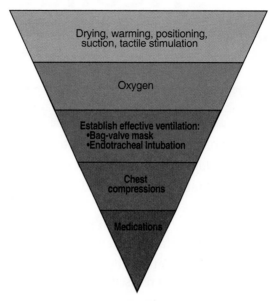

Figure 8-1. The inverted pyramid reflects the relative frequency of various steps in neonatal resuscitation.

PREPARATION FOR DELIVERY

Factors Associated with Increased Risk for Neonatal Resuscitation - **Antepartum**

1. Maternal age > 35 years or <16 years
2. Maternal diabetes
3. Maternal hemorrhage
4. Maternal drug therapy - magnesium, adrenergic-blocking drugs, lithium carbonate
5. Maternal substance abuse - heroin, methadone
6. Previous fetal or neonatal death
7. No prenatal care
8. Chronic or pregnancy-induce hypertension
9. Maternal anemia or isoimmunication
10. Fetal malformation identified by ultrasound
11. Premature rupture of membranes
12. Preterm/postterm fetus
13. Small fetus for dates
14. Oligohydramnios
15. Multiple fetuses
16. Maternal illness
17. Immature pulmonary studies

Factors Associated with Increased Risk for Neonatal Resuscitation - **Intrapartum**	1. Abnormal presentation

Factors Associated with Increased Risk for Neonatal Resuscitation - **Intrapartum**

1. Abnormal presentation
2. Infection
3. Prolonged labor
4. Prolonged rupture of membranes
5. Prolapsed cord
6. Heavy sedation of mother
7. Meconium-stained fluid
8. Indexes of fetal distress (fetal heart rate abnormalities)
9. Operative delivery
10. Profuse bleeding
11. Precipitous labor
12. Foul-smelling amniotic fluid
13. Abnormal fetal heart rate

Body Substance Isolation Precautions

1. Body substance isolation precautions are particularly important in the delivery area due to the likelihood of exposure to blood and other body fluids.

PERSONNEL

1. At least one person skilled in newborn resuscitation should attend every delivery.
2. Additional trained persons should be readily available.
   a. Resuscitation of a severely depressed newborn requires at least two people - one to ventilate (and intubate if necessary), the other to monitor and perform chest compressions if required.
   b. Should it become necessary, a third person is desirable to insert intravascular catheters and administer medications.

TEMPERATURE REGULATION

Heat loss may be prevented by:

1. Removing wet linens from contact with the infant
2. Placing the neonate under a preheated warmer or heat lamps
3. Quickly drying the amniotic fluid covering the newborn

INITIAL STABILIZATION

POSITIONING

1. Dry the newborn quickly and place supine or on his/her side with the neck in a neutral position.
    a. Overextension or flexion of the neck may produce airway obstruction.
    b. Proper head position may be helped by placing a blanket or towel (approximately 1 inch thick) under the newborn's shoulders.
2. If copious secretions are present, place the infant on his/her side with the neck slightly extended.

SUCTIONING

1. After delivery of the head (but before delivery of the shoulders), the mouth of the newborn should be suctioned with a bulb syringe, and then the nose.
2. Suctioning should be limited to 3-5 seconds at a time.
    a. **Monitor the heart rate for possible bradycardia.**
    b. Deep suctioning of the oropharynx may stimulate the vagus nerve resulting in bradycardia and/or apnea.
3. Ventilate with 100% oxygen between suctioning attempts.

TACTILE STIMULATION

1. Effective respirations are induced in most newborns through the stimulation received during drying, warming, and suctioning.
2. Methods recommended for providing additional stimulation, if needed, are:
   a. Flicking the soles of the feet
   b. Rubbing the back
3. **Positive-pressure ventilation should be initiated if there is no response to tactile stimulation after a brief (5-10 second) period of stimulation.**

EVALUATION

Evaluation begins during the process of initial stabilization with assessment of:
- Respiratory effort
- Heart rate
- Color

1. Respiratory effort - crying, adequate respirations, gasping, apneic
   - The term infant's respiratory rate is normally between 30 and 60 breaths/minute in the first 12 hours of life
2. Heart rate may be evaluated by:
   a. Listening to the apical beat with a stethoscope
   b. Feeling the pulse by lightly grasping the base of the umbilical cord
   c. Palpation of the brachial or femoral pulse
      - The term infant's heart rate is normally 100-180 beats/minute in the first 12 hours of life
3. Color - evaluate for central cyanosis
   a. Acrocyanosis (cyanosis of the extremities) is common and does not reflect inadequate oxygenation
   b. Pallor may indicate decreased cardiac output, severe anemia, hypothermia, acidosis, or hypovolemia

Apgar Scoring System

Resuscitation of the newborn should not be delayed to obtain an Apgar score

1. The Apgar scoring system is a numerical method of rating the condition of the neonate after birth.

2. The five objective signs are evaluated at 1 and 5 minutes after birth.

    a. A score of 0, 1 or 2 is given for each of the five signs assessed. The minimum Apgar score is 0 and the maximum is 10.

    b. If the Apgar score at 5 minutes is less than 7, additional scores are obtained every 5 minutes for a total of 20 minutes.

3. **The Apgar score should not be used to determine the need for resuscitation.**

4. Scoring:

    *   0 - 3 indicates a neonate in severe distress

    *   4 - 6 indicates a moderately distressed neonate

    *   7 - 10 indicates a mildly distressed neonate or one with no distress

Table 8-1. The Apgar Scoring System.

Sign	0	1	2
Appearance (Skin color)	Blue, pale	Body pink, blue extremities	Completely pink
Pulse Rate (Heart rate)	Absent	< 100/minute	> 100/minute
Grimace (Irritability)	No response	Grimace	Cough, sneeze, cry
Activity (Muscle tone)	Limp	Some flexion	Active motion
Respirations (Respiratory effort)	Absent	Slow, irregular	Good, crying

OXYGEN ADMINISTRATION

Free-flow oxygen - blowing oxygen over the neonate's nose to enhance breathing of oxygen-enriched air

1. Early administration of 100% oxygen is important if signs of neonatal distress are present during the initial steps of stabilization (cyanosis, bradycardia or other signs of distress).

2. Oxygen can initially be delivered by free-flow through a face mask (applied **firmly** to the face) connected to an anesthesia bag.

   a. If a mask is not available, use a funnel attached to oxygen supply tubing and an oxygen source set to deliver at least 5 liters/minute or cup the hand with oxygen tubing around the neonate's face to maximize the concentration of oxygen to the mouth and nose.

   b. Optimal oxygen concentrations (about 80%) can be delivered with the oxygen tubing placed approximately 1/2 inch from the nose. Oxygen concentration rapidly declines as the distance between the oxygen tubing and face increases.

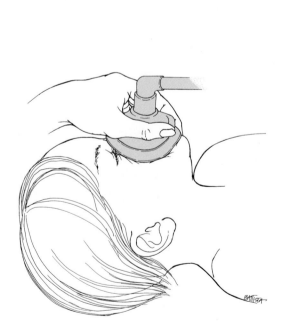

Figure 8-2. Administering oxygen via face mask for the neonate.

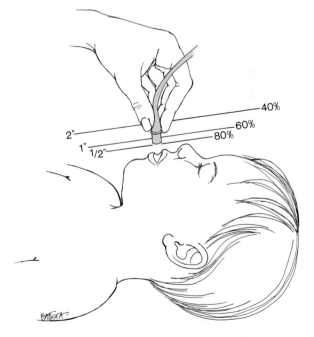

Figure 8-3. Administering oxygen via oxygen tubing for the neonate.

3. The risks of administering too much oxygen during the brief interval needed for resuscitation should not cause concern.

4. Enough oxygen must be provided for the infant to become pink. If oxygen is to be administered for more than a few minutes, it should be heated and humidified to prevent heat loss and drying of the respiratory mucosa.[1]

VENTILATION

Indications for Positive-Pressure Ventilation

Most neonates requiring ventilatory support may be adequately ventilated using a bag and mask.

Indications for positive-pressure ventilation:

- Apnea or gasping respirations
- Heart rate less than 100 beats/minute
- Persistent central cyanosis despite administration of 100% oxygen

Assisting Ventilation

1. Respirations should be assisted at a rate of 40-60 breaths per minute

2. Pressures of 30-40 cm H_2O or higher may be needed to provide initial lung inflation. Less pressure is usually needed for subsequent breaths.

3. Signs of adequate ventilation include:
   a. Bilateral chest compressions
   b. Presence of bilateral breath sounds
   c. Improvement in color and heart rate

4. If the lungs do not inflate adequately:
   a. Reposition the face mask
   b. Reposition the head
   c. Assess for secretions and suction if necessary
   d. Consider increasing inflation pressure
      - If these maneuvers are not successful in providing adequate ventilation, immediate endotracheal intubation and ventilation are required.

5. Bag-mask ventilation may produce gastric distention.

    a. If bag-valve-mask ventilation is necessary for more than approximately 2 minutes, or if gastric distention develops, insert an 8 or 10F orogastric tube and leave it open to air. Aspirate periodically with a 20-ml syringe.[2]

      • Proper length of the inserted catheter is determined by measuring the distance from the bridge of the nose to the earlobe plus the distance from the earlobe to the xiphoid process.[4]

    b. Larger tubes may interfere with obtaining a proper seal between the face and mask.

6. After adequate ventilation has been instituted for 15-30 seconds, evaluate the heart rate.

    a. If the heart rate is < 60 beats/min or between 60 and 80 beats/min and not increasing, continue assisted ventilation and initiate chest compressions.

    b. If the heart rate is 60-80 beats/min and increasing, continue assisted ventilation. Chest compressions are not necessary.

    c. If the heart rate is at least 100 beats/minute and spontaneous respirations are present, the rate and pressure of assisted ventilation may be reduced gradually.

      • Observe the neonate for signs of adequate spontaneous respiration before ceasing ventilation.

      • Gentle tactile stimulation may help maintain spontaneous breathing.

      • Continue assisted ventilation if spontaneous respirations are inadequate.

A poor response to ventilation efforts may be the result of:

1. A poor seal between the face and mask

2. Poor alignment of the head and neck

3. Insufficient ventilating pressure

4. Improper endotracheal tube position

SELF-INFLATING BAGS

Description

1. Self-inflating bags refill independent of gas flow when the grip on the bag is released.

2. To deliver high concentrations of oxygen (90-100%) with this device, supplemental oxygen and an oxygen reservoir must be used.

Pop-Off Valves

1. Some self-inflating bags are equipped with a pop-off (pressure-release) valve that is set to release at 30-45 cm H_2O, preventing pressure from being delivered to the neonate.

2. To effectively deliver ventilations to a neonate, higher pressures than those of the preset limits of the pop-off valve may be needed, especially with the first few breaths.

3. Self-inflating bags without a pop-off valve, or self-inflating bags with a bypassed pop-off valve, should have a pressure gauge attached to the self-inflating bag.

4. Use a self-inflating bag with a volume of 450 ml.

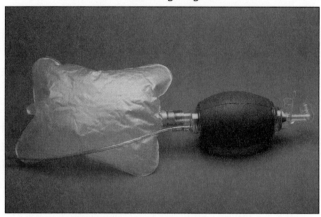

Figure 8-4. Self-inflating bag.

ANESTHESIA (FLOW-INFLATING) BAG

1. The anesthesia bag inflates only when air or oxygen is forced into it. The bag is kept inflated when a tight seal is made between the mask and the neonate's face.

2. A pressure gauge must be present when using this device since anesthesia bags can deliver very high pressures.

3. Provides more reliable control of oxygen concentration and a greater range in peak inspiratory pressures than the self-inflating bag.

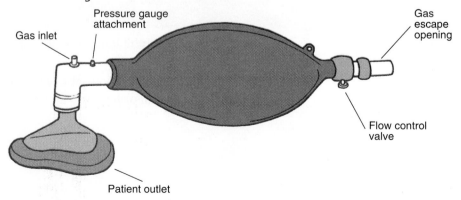

Figure 8-5. Anesthesia bag.

FACE MASKS

Face masks are available in a variety of shapes and sizes. The preferred mask is one that has a cushioned rim and is anatomically shaped. This type of mask offers several advantages:

1. Low dead space (< 5 ml)
2. Less pressure required to maintain a tight seal than with round or noncushioned masks
3. Less chance of injury to the neonate's eyes if the mask is improperly positioned

A correctly sized mask avoids the eyes and covers the nose, mouth and tip of the chin. Masks fitting preterm, term and large newborns should be available.

ENDOTRACHEAL INTUBATION

Indications

1. When bag-mask ventilation is ineffective as evidenced by:
   a. Inadequate chest expansion
   b. Persistent low heart rate
2. When tracheal suctioning is required, especially for thick meconium
3. When prolonged positive-pressure ventilation is necessary or anticipated.
4. When diaphragmatic hernia is suspected.

Endotracheal Tubes

The length of the endotracheal tube should be of uniform internal diameter - not tapered near the distal tip.

Vocal Cord Guide

1. Most neonatal endotracheal tubes have a vocal cord line (a black line near the distal tip of the endotracheal tube).
2. The tip of the endotracheal tube should be inserted until the vocal cord guide is at the level of the cords. In this position, the tip of the endotracheal tube should lie approximately half-way between the vocal cords and carina.

Endotracheal Tube Size

1. A guide to deciding proper distance for insertion of the endotracheal tube is the "tip-to-lip" measurement.

   6 + infant's weight in kg = distance (in cm) from the tip of the tube to the infant's lips

2. ET tube size in mm = $\dfrac{\text{postconceptual age in weeks}}{10}$

Table 8-2. Endotracheal Tube Size.

Tube Size (mm ID)	Weight	Gestational Age
2.5	< 1000 g	< 28 weeks
3.0	1000-2000 g	28-34 weeks
3.5	2000-3000 g	34-38 weeks
3.5-4.0	> 3000 g	> 38 weeks

Source: Bloom, R (ed), *Textbook of Neonatal Resuscitation.* Dallas: American Heart Association, 1994.

Confirming Tube Placement	1. Watch for symmetrical rise and fall of the chest.
	2. Listen high in the axillae for equal breath sounds and absent sounds over the stomach
	3. Confirm there is no gastric distention with ventilation
	4. Note improvement in color, heart rate and activity
	5. Note the exhaled carbon dioxide level
	6. Obtain chest x-ray for final confirmation of tube placement
Complications	1. Hypoxia
	2. Infection
	3. Pneumothorax
	4. Bradycardia, apnea
	5. Perforation of the trachea or esophagus
	6. Trauma to the lips, tongue, gums, trachea, vocal cords, esophagus

CHEST COMPRESSIONS

Indications

Chest compressions are indicated in the neonate if, after 15-30 seconds of positive-pressure ventilation with 100% oxygen:

1. The heart rate is < 60 beats/minute or
2. The heart rate is between 60 and 80 beats/minute and **NOT** rapidly increasing.

Preferred Method - Thumb Technique	1. The thumbs are placed on the middle 1/3 of the sternum, just below the nipple line, encircling the chest with both hands. The fingers are used to support the neonate's back.
	2. The thumbs are placed side by side unless the neonate is small, in which case the thumbs may be placed one over the other.
	3. Compress the chest 1/2 to 3/4 inch while another rescuer ventilates.
	4. Check for a pulse after 30 seconds.
	a. If the heart rate is less than 80 beats/min, continue chest compressions and positive-pressure ventilation.
	b. If the heart rate is 80/min or above, stop chest compressions. Continue positive-pressure ventilation until the heart rate is > 100 beats/min and the infant is breathing spontaneously.
Two-Finger Method	If the infant is large or the hands of the rescuer are small, use the infant CPR technique.
Compression-Ventilation Ratio	1. Chest compressions should be interposed with ventilations in a ratio of 3:1.
	2. The combined rate of compressions and ventilations should be 120 per minute (90 compressions, 30 breaths).
	3. The compressor should pause after each third compression to allow delivery of an effective breath. It is helpful for the compressor to count aloud, "One-and-two-and-three-and-bag-and..."

MEDICATIONS

Indications	Bradycardia in the neonate is usually the result of profound hypoxia.
	Medications are indicated when the infant's heart rate remains below 80 despite adequate ventilation (with 100% oxygen) and chest compressions.

ROUTES OF ADMINISTRATION

Umbilical Vein	1. Preferred means of vascular access during neonatal resuscitation:
	• Easily located
	• Easily cannulated

2. Anatomy

    a. Two arteries and one vein readily identified in the umbilical cord stump

    b. The vein is a thin-walled, single vessel

    c. The arteries are thicker-walled, paired and often constricted.

3. Cannulation

    a. A 3.5 of 5.0F umbilical catheter is attached to a 3-way stopcock and filled with saline

    b. The catheter is inserted into the vein until the tip of the catheter is just below the skin and there is free flow of blood

        *   Inserting the catheter a further distance than recommended increases the risk of infusing solutions into the liver

        *   If possible, the catheter should be removed at the end of the resuscitation to reduce the risk of infection or portal vein thrombosis.

4. Complications

    *   Infection

    *   Embolism

    *   Portal vein thrombosis

Peripheral Venous Access

Veins of the scalp and extremities are acceptable routes for administration of fluids and medications but are difficult to access during resuscitation of the neonate.

Endotracheal Administration

If vascular access is not available, epinephrine and naloxone may be administered endotracheally. Endotracheal dose is the same as the IV dose.

1. Insert a 5F feeding tube through the endotracheal tube.

2. Dilute drug with 3-5 ml of normal saline and administer into the feeding tube.

3. Flush the feeding tube with approximately 0.5 ml of normal saline.

4. Remove the feeding tube.

5. Provide several positive-pressure ventilations to distribute the drug throughout the bronchial tree.

DRUG	MECHANISM OF ACTION/EFFECTS	INDICATIONS	DOSAGE
Epinephrine Trade Name: Adrenalin	Produces beneficial effects in patients during cardiac arrest primarily because of its alpha-adrenergic stimulating properties Alpha-adrenergic effects: Increases peripheral vascular resistance (vasoconstriction) → increases diastolic pressure → increases myocardial and cerebral blood flow during CPR Beta-adrenergic effects: • Increased heart rate (+ chronotropy) • Increased myocardial contractility (+ inotropy) • Increased automaticity (+ dromotropy) • Results in increased myocardial oxygen consumption	Asystole Spontaneous heart rate of < 80 beats/min despite adequate ventilation with 100% oxygen and chest compressions	May be administered IV, IO, or ET 0.01 to 0.03 mg/kg (0.1-0.3 ml/kg) of 1:10,000 solution May be repeated every 3-5 minutes If no response to ET administration, may increase dose up to 0.1 mg/kg (0.1 ml/kg of 1:1000) High-dose epi (10x) not routinely recommended, may potentiate intracranial bleeding
Naloxone Trade Name: Narcan Class: Narcotic Antagonist	Competes with opiod receptor sites in the central nervous system, displacing previously administered narcotic analgesics	Reversal of respiratory depression in the newborn induced by narcotics administered to the mother within 4 hours of delivery Avoid if mother is addicted to narcotics. Administration of naloxone to these infants may induce a withdrawal reaction.	May be administered IV, IO, ET, IM, SQ 0.1 mg/kg Repeat administration of naloxone may be needed since the duration of action of narcotics may exceed that of naloxone

VOLUME EXPANDERS

Indications	Class I (definitely helpful) when there is evidence or suspicion of acute bleeding with signs of hypovolemia.
Signs of Hypovolemia[3]	1. Pallor persisting after oxygenation 2. Weak pulses with a **good** heart rate 3. Poor response to resuscitative efforts 4. Decreased blood pressure (may not be available)
Types of Volume Expanders	1. Normal saline or Ringer's lactate 2. 5% albumin or other plasma substitute 3. O-negative blood crossmatched with the mother's blood
Dosage	10 ml/kg administered over 5-10 minutes Repeat if signs of hypovolemia are present

SPECIAL CONSIDERATIONS

MECONIUM-STAINED AMNIOTIC FLUID

Meconium Aspiration Syndrome (MAS)

Significant cause of neonatal morbidity and mortality

Includes:

1. Respiratory distress with cyanosis in room air
2. Aspiration pneumonia
3. Pneumothorax
4. Pulmonary hypertension (severe cases)

Newborns at Risk

1. Those most at risk are newborns delivered through thick, particulate meconium.
2. A milder form of meconium aspiration syndrome can occur when the fluid is thin.
3. 20-30% of neonates will have meconium in the trachea despite thorough suctioning of the nose, mouth and posterior pharynx before delivery of the shoulders and thorax.
   - Suggests a significant incidence of in-utero aspiration

Suctioning

1. Suctioning of the mouth, nose and posterior pharynx should be performed before delivery of the shoulders and again after delivery when the infant has been placed on a radiant warmer in all neonates with meconium staining.
   - Use of a large-bore (12 to 14F) catheter is recommended, although a bulb syringe may be adequate.
2. If the meconium is thick and particulate, or the infant is depressed, direct endotracheal suctioning should be performed.
   a. The endotracheal tube is used as a suction catheter and suction is applied as the tube is slowly withdrawn.
   b. The procedure should be repeated until the meconium clears.
      - Suction catheters should not be passed through the endotracheal tube for initial removal of meconium particulate.
      - Once the meconium is cleared, a suction catheter may be passed through the endotracheal tube for subsequent suctioning.

3. In the severely depressed newborn, positive-pressure ventilation should be considered, even if the trachea has not been completely cleared of meconium.

4. The stomach should be suctioned after the infant is stabilized to prevent possible aspiration of gastric contents containing meconium.

PRETERM NEWBORNS

Anticipation

Mobilize specially trained personnel and equipment

Heat Loss

Preterm infants are more susceptible to heat loss than term neonates due to:

- Thin epidermis
- High ratio of surface area to body mass
- Insufficiently developed temperature control mechanism
- Inability to shiver

Methods of reducing heat loss:

1. Prewarm radiant warmer, towels and blankets
2. Maintain a warm delivery room
3. Consider covering the infant with a thin layer of clear plastic sheeting

Airway Management

Preterm infants have an increased need for assisted ventilation due to diminished lung compliance, respiratory musculature and respiratory drive.

"Some experts believe that the extremely preterm neonates should be electively intubated and ventilated rather than given a trial of spontaneous ventilation assisted by bag and mask."[7]

Medications

1. The brain of the preterm infant is vulnerable to bleeding when subjected to rapid changes in vascular pressure and osmolarity.
2. Minimize the use of rapid boluses of volume expanders or hyperosmolar solutions, such as sodium bicarbonate.

REFERENCES

1. Bloom R (ed.), *Textbook of Neonatal Resuscitation.* Dallas: American Heart Association, 1994.

2. Chameides L., Hazinski MF (ed.), *Textbook of Pediatric Advanced Life Support.* Dallas: American Heart Association, 1994, p. 9-5.

3. Chameides L., Hazinski MF (ed.), *Textbook of Pediatric Advanced Life Support.* Dallas: American Heart Association, 1994, p. 9-8.

QUIZ – POSTRESUSCITATION STABILIZATION AND NEONATAL RESUSCITATION

1. During resuscitation, the neonate should be placed:

   a. prone or on his/her side with the neck in a neutral position
   b. supine or on his/her side with the neck in a neutral position
   c. supine in a slight Trendelenburg position with the neck slightly extended
   d. on his/her side in a slight Trendelenburg position with the neck slightly extended

2. Which of the following are indicators of end-organ perfusions?
   1. mental status, 2. capillary refill, 3. pulse quality

   a. 1, 2
   b. 1, 3
   c. 2, 3
   d. 1, 2, 3

3. Evaluation of the newborn begins during initial stabilization. Which of the following correctly reflects the clinical signs to be evaluated?

   a. respiratory effort, heart rate, color
   b. heart rate, respiratory effort, activity
   c. respiratory effort, heart rate, muscle tone
   d. color, respiratory effort, reflex irritability

4. The neonate's chest should be compressed _____ at a rate of _____.

   a. 1/2 to 1 inch, 100 beats/minute
   b. 1/2 to 1 inch, 120 beats/minute
   c. 1/2 to 3/4 inch, 100 beats/minute
   d. 1/2 to 3/4 inch, 120 beats/minute

5. A 6 lb. 6 1/2 oz. baby girl has been delivered vaginally. The infant has been suctioned, positioned, warmed, and stimulated but remains apneic. Chest expansion does not occur despite attempts to ventilate with a bag-mask device. What should be done now?

   _____

   _____

   _____

6. Which of the following is the preferred route for administration of medications during neonatal resuscitation?

   a. scalp vein
   b. endotracheal
   c. umbilical vein
   d. intracardiac injection

7. The recommended initial neonatal dose of naloxone is:

   a.   10 ml/kg
   b.   1 mEq/kg
   c.   0.1 mg/kg
   d.   0.01 mg/kg

8. Care must be taken to minimize the use of rapid boluses of volume expanders or hyperosmolar solutions, such as sodium bicarbonate, when administering medications to a preterm infant because portions of the brain are particularly vulnerable to bleeding when subjected to rapid changes in vascular pressure and osmolarity.

   a.   true
   b.   false

9. List five (5) clinical signs of inadequate systemic perfusion.

   1.   _____

   2.   _____

   3.   _____

   4.   _____

   5.   _____

10. Assessment of a newborn one minute after delivery reveals the infant to be crying vigorously upon light flicking of the foot. The heart rate is 130 beats/minute and some flexion of the extremities is noted. Respirations are regular at approximately 40 breaths/minute. The body is pink and the extremities blue. You would assign an Apgar score of:

    a.   7
    b.   8
    c.   9
    d.   10

11. The initial rate of mechanical or manual ventilation should be __ breaths/minute for infants and __ breaths/minute for older children.

    a.   16-20, 20-30
    b.   20-30, 16-20
    c.   40-60, 16-20
    d.   40-60, 20-30

12. Correct placement of an endotracheal tube should result in all of the following EXCEPT:

    a.   bilateral, equal breath sounds
    b.   symmetrical chest wall motion
    c.   absence of abdominal distention
    d.   presence of sounds over the stomach

13. Volume expansion should begin with an initial bolus of ___ in a neonate, ___ in an infant or child, of normal saline or lactated Ringer's solution.

   a. 10 ml/kg, 10 ml/kg
   b. 10 ml/kg, 20 ml/kg
   c. 20 ml/kg, 20 ml/kg
   d. 20 ml/kg, 30 ml/kg

14. Suctioning of the neonate should be limited to _____ seconds at a time.

   a. 3-5
   b. 5-10
   c. 10-15
   d. 15-30

15. Acceptable methods of stimulating the newborn include:

   a. rubbing the back, slapping or flicking the soles of the feet
   b. slapping or flicking the soles of the feet, squeezing the rib cage
   c. blowing cold air or oxygen onto the face or body, rubbing the back
   d. squeezing the rib cage, blowing cold air or oxygen onto the face or body

16. A neonate has been ventilated with 100% oxygen for 30 seconds. The heart rate is 70 beats/minute and chest compressions are initiated. After 30 seconds of chest compressions and positive-pressure ventilation, the heart rate is now 90 beats/minute and spontaneous respirations are present. What action should be taken at this time?

   a. discontinue chest compressions and positive-pressure ventilation
   b. discontinue chest compressions and continue positive-pressure ventilation
   c. continue chest compressions and positive-pressure ventilation until the heart rate is at least 100 beats/minute
   d. discontinue positive-pressure ventilation and continue chest compressions until the heart rate is at least 100 beats/minute

17. When providing free-flow oxygen during resuscitation of a neonate, the oxygen flowmeter should be set to deliver at least _____ liters/minute.

   a. 5
   b. 8
   c. 10
   d. 15

18. List two (2) methods that may be used to reduce heat loss in the newborn.

   1. _____

   2. _____

19. List two (2) conditions that may produce unilateral breath sounds.

1. _____

2. _____

20. Signs of hypovolemia in the neonate include:
1. Weak pulses with a good heart rate
2. Pallor persisting after oxygenation
3. Poor response to resuscitative efforts

a. 1, 2
b. 2, 3
c. 1, 3
d. 1, 2, 3

QUIZ ANSWERS – POSTRESUSCITATION STABILIZATION AND NEONATAL RESUSCITATION

QUESTION	ANSWER	RATIONALE	STUDY GUIDE REFERENCE	PALS PAGE REFERENCE
1	B	During resuscitation, the neonate should be placed supine or on his/her side with the neck in a neutral position.	190	9-3
2	D	Signs of end-organ perfusion that should be evaluated include mental status, capillary refill, and pulse quality (blood pressure), skin temperature, urine output.	183	10-3, 10-4
3	A	Evaluation of the newborn begins during the process of initial stabilization with assessment of respiratory effort, heart rate and color (in that order).	191	9-4
4	D	The neonate's chest should be compressed 1/2 to 3/4 inch at a rate of 120 beats/minute.	199	9-6
5		Reposition the mask, reposition the head, check for secretions and suction if necessary, increase ventilation pressure. If these measures do not provide adequate ventilation, immediate endotracheal intubation and ventilation is required.	194	9-5
6	C	During neonatal resuscitation, the umbilical vein is the preferred method of vascular access for administration of fluids and medications since it is easily located and large enough to be cannulated rapidly.	199	9-7

7	C	The recommended initial dose of naloxone is 0.1 mg/kg IV, IO, ET or, if perfusion is adequate, IM or SQ. This dose may be repeated every 2-3 minutes as needed.	201	9-8
8	A	True. The anatomy of the brain of the preterm infant includes a fragile subependymal germinal matrix, which is particularly vulnerable to bleeding when subjected to rapid changes in vascular pressure and osmolarity.	203	9-9
9		Signs of inadequate systemic perfusion include hypotension, delayed capillary refill, absence or decreased intensity of peripheral pulses, altered mental status, cool extremities, decreased urine output and tachycardia.	183	10-4
10	B	An Apgar score of 8 is assigned based on the following: Some flexion of the extremities (1 point) Regular respirations (2 points) Blue extremities, pink body (1 point) Heart rate > 100 (2 points) Vigorous crying on stimulation (2 points)	192	9-5
11	B	The initial rate of mechanical or manual ventilation should be **20-30** breaths/minute for infants, **16-20** breaths/minute for older children.	181	10-3

12	D	Correct endotracheal tube position should be checked by: 1. Watching for symmetrical chest wall motion 2. Listening for equal breath sounds high in the axillae and for **absence** of sounds over the stomach 3. Checking for absence of abdominal distention with positive-pressure ventillation 4. Noting improvement in color, heart rate and activity of the neonate 5. Chest X-ray 6. Noting the exhaled CO_2 level, if available	198	9-7
13	B	Volume expansion in the neonate should begin with an initial fluid bolus of 10 ml/kg, 20 ml/kg in the infant or child.	140, 202	6-2, 9-8
14	A	Suctioning of the neonate should be limited to 3-5 seconds at a time.	191	9-4
15	A	Acceptable methods of providing tactile stimulation to the newborn include flicking or slapping the soles of the feet and rubbing the back.	191	9-4
16	B	Continue positive-pressure ventilation but discontinue chest compressions. When the heart rate reaches 100 beats/minute or above, the rate and pressure of assisted positive-pressure ventilation should be reduced **gradually** while the infant is observed for signs of adequate spontaneous respiration.	195	9-7

17	A	When providing free-flow oxygen by means of oxygen tubing or face mask, the oxygen flowmeter should be set to deliver at least **5** liters/minute.	193	9-6
18		Methods used to minimize heat loss in the newborn include: 1. Placing the infant under a preheated warmer or heat lamps 2. Quickly drying the infant of amniotic fluid 3. Removing wet linens from contact with the infant	190	9-2
19		Right mainstem bronchus intubation may produce unilateral breath sounds on the right. Unilateral breath sounds may also be due to pneumothorax, mucous plug, pleural effusion, lung consolidation or foreign body obstruction.	182	9-6
20	D	Signs of hypovolemia in the neonate include pallor persisting after oxygenation, weak pulses with a **good** heart rate, poor response to resuscitative efforts and decreased blood pressure.	201	9-8

Posttest

1. Systemic complications of intravascular access include:
   a. phlebitis
   b. cellulitis
   c. hematoma formation
   d. catheter-fragment embolism

2. Which of the following is least likely to be associated with obstruction of the lower airway?
   a. stridor
   b. wheezing
   c. retractions
   d. nasal flaring

A seven month old is brought in pulseless and apneic. CPR is in progress. An endotracheal tube is quickly placed and placement is confirmed by the presence of equal bilateral breath sounds and good chest rise. The infant is being hyperventilated with 100% oxygen and CPR is continuing. The cardiac monitor displays the following rhythm:

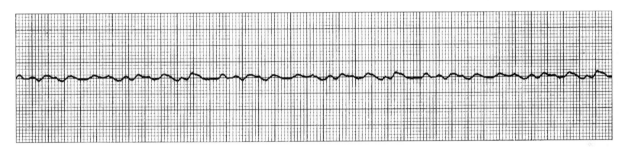

Figure 9-1.

3. The rhythm displayed above is: _____

4. Which of the following interventions should be done next?
   a. defibrillate up to three times if needed
   b. obtain intravenous or intraosseous access
   c. administer lidocaine 1 mg/kg endotracheally
   d. administer epinephrine 0.01 mg/kg endotracheally

5. Naloxone:
   a. is a volume expander
   b. is a narcotic antagonist
   c. increases heart rate and myocardial contractility
   d. may correct acidosis by raising the pH of the blood

6. A child with signs of cyanosis, diminished breath sounds with minimal chest excursion, and an inadequate respiratory rate is exhibiting signs of:
   a. hypothermia
   b. hypovolemia
   c. respiratory failure
   d. early respiratory distress

7. Complications that may occur in the pediatric patient with the use of an oxygen-powered breathing device include:

    1. gastric distention
    2. esophageal perforation
    3. tension pneumothorax
    4. pleural infection

    a. 1, 3
    b. 2, 4
    c. 3, 4
    d. 1, 2, 3

8. Nearly 1/2 of all pediatric injuries and deaths are the result of:

    a. burns
    b. submersion
    c. firearm injuries
    d. motor vehicle-related trauma

9. Primary causes of circulatory failure in children include:

    1. Sepsis
    2. Fluid loss due to burns, vomiting
    3. Epiglottitis
    4. Heart rate abnormalities
    5. Foreign body airway obstruction

    a. 3, 5
    b. 1, 2
    c. 1, 2, 4
    d. 2, 3, 5

10. Attempts to intubate an infant or child should not exceed __ seconds and the heart rate should be monitored during the procedure.

    a. 5
    b. 10
    c. 15
    d. 30

11. Crystalloid solutions:

    a. are inexpensive
    b. have a short shelf-life
    c. are likely to cause adverse reactions
    d. are efficient in rapidly expanding the intravascular compartment

12. Cessation of ventilation and circulation most often results in:

    a. metabolic alkalosis

    b. respiratory alkalosis

    c. a mixed metabolic and respiratory acidosis

    d. a mixed metabolic and respiratory alkalosis

13. When ventricular fibrillation is present in a child, one should search for a metabolic abnormality (calcium, potassium, magnesium or glucose imbalances), hypothermia or drug toxicity (digitalis or cyclic antidepressants).

    a. true

    b. false

14. Which of the following may be administered intravenously, endotracheally and by intraosseous infusion?

    1. Epinephrine

    2. Lidocaine

    3. Sodium bicarbonate

    4. Naloxone

    5. Dopamine

    a. 1, 2, 3

    b. 1, 2, 4

    c. 3, 4, 5

    d. 1, 3, 5

15. Bretylium may be beneficial in the treatment of:

    a. bradycardia

    b. pulseless electrical activity

    c. refractory supraventricular tachycardia

    d. refractory ventricular fibrillation or pulseless ventricular tachycardia

16. Complications of central venous cannulation include:

    a. infection, aspiration

    b. osteomyelitis, air embolism

    c. infection, air embolism, pneumothorax

    d. osteomyelitis, aspiration, pneumothorax

17. Which of the following cardiovascular effects can be expected from epinephrine in the dose used during resuscitation?

    a. increased heart rate, decreased cardiac output

    b. increased heart rate, increased systemic vascular resistance

    c. decreased systemic vascular resistance, increased heart rate

    d. decreased automaticity, increased myocardial contractility

18. Explain the mechanism by which rapid heart rates may adversely affect cardiac output.

_____

_____

_____

19. Verapamil:

    a. is not recommended for use in the pediatric patient
    b. is the drug of choice in the treatment of symptomatic bradycardia
    c. is the drug of choice in the treatment of supraventricular tachycardia
    d. should be administered before defibrillation attempts in pulseless ventricular tachycardia

20. Describe the ECG characteristics of ventricular tachycardia.

    Rate: _____

    Rhythm: _____

    P waves: _____

    QRS: _____

    T waves: _____

21. The recommended endotracheal tube size for a 6 year old is:

    a. 4.0
    b. 5.5
    c. 6.5
    d. 7.0

22. Delivery of high concentrations of oxygen with a self-inflating bag requires an attached oxygen reservoir.

    a. true
    b. false

23. Sodium bicarbonate:

    1. may result in severe dysrhythmias in patients on digitalis
    2. is sclerosing to small veins
    3. may be administered endotracheally in the same dose used IV
    4. produces a chemical burn if extravasation occurs

    a. 1, 2   c. 3, 4
    b. 2, 4   d. 1, 3

24. Paramedics are en route to your facility with a 3-year old submersion victim. While awaiting the arrival of this patient, estimate the following:

   a. Weight in kilograms _____
   b. Endotracheal tube size _____
   c. Normal systolic blood pressure _____
   d. Normal heart rate _____
   e. Normal respiratory rate _____

25. Explain the significance of the inverted pyramid in neonatal resuscitation.

   _____

   _____

26. Which of the following statements is correct regarding pediatric CPR?

   a. the compression-ventilation ratio is 3:1 in the neonate
   b. the compression-ventilation ratio is 15:2 for single-rescuer CPR in the child
   c. the chest should be depressed 1/2 to 3/4 inch in the neonate using the heel of the rescuer's hand
   d. ventilations should be delivered at a rate of 40-60 per minute for single-rescuer CPR in the child

27. You are called to evaluate a three month old brought in to the Emergency Department by an anxious mother. Evaluation reveals the infant to be cyanotic and lethargic. The respiratory rate is 48 and rales are heard bilaterally on auscultation. Intercostal retractions are noted. The extremities are cool and capillary refill is three seconds. You are unable to palpate distal pulses and the femoral pulse is too fast to count. Describe your immediate course of action.

   _____

   _____

   The infant's condition remains unchanged despite your initial interventions. The cardiac monitor reveals the rhythm below:

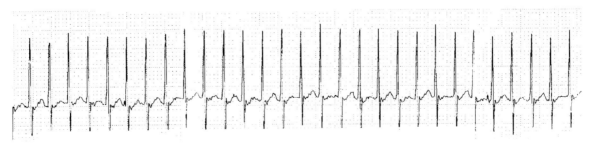

Figure 9-2.

28. a. Recalling the three categories of pediatric rhythms, this rhythm is categorized as a(n) _____ rhythm.
    b. Is the infant stable or unstable? _____

29. The infant's condition remains unchanged despite administration of high concentration oxygen. An IV has been successfully placed. Which of the following reflects the most appropriate course of action at this time?

    a. defibrillate immediately with 3 stacked countershocks of 2 joules/kg, 4 joules/kg and 4 joules/kg
    b. administer adenosine 0.1 mg/kg or perform synchronized countershock with 0.5 joules/kg
    c. administer verapamil 0.1 mg/kg or perform synchronized countershock with 0.5 joules/kg
    d. administer lidocaine 1 mg/kg and defibrillate with 2 joules/kg within 30-60 seconds of lidocaine administration

30. A 27 year old pregnant female arrives in the Emergency Department stating her baby is "coming now." Questioning reveals her due date to have been one week ago. Moments later the amniotic sac breaks and inspection of the perineum reveals a crowning infant. Thick meconium is evident. Describe how you will manage this situation.

    _____

    _____

31. A five month old infant is brought to the Emergency Department with a two-day history of vomiting and diarrhea. Examination of the infant reveals equal chest rise with clear, bilateral breath sounds and a respiratory rate of 40/minute. The extremities are cool and dry. Capillary refill is 3-4 seconds. The mucous membranes appear dry. Distal pulses are weak; the heart rate is approximately 150 beats/minute. The infant will not take a bottle.

    Is this infant in respiratory failure or shock? _____

32. Describe your initial management priorities in the treatment of this patient.

    _____

    _____

33. Which of the following statements is **INCORRECT** regarding dopamine?

    a. The recommended dosage range for dopamine administration is 2-20 mcg/kg/minute.
    b. Dopamine has a short plasma half-life and must be administered by constant infusion.
    c. Dopamine suppresses ventricular ectopy and elevates the ventricular fibrillation threshold.
    d. Dopamine is indicated in the treatment of circulatory shock following resuscitation or when shock is unresponsive to fluid administration.

34. Resuscitation bags used for ventilation of full-term neonates, infants and children should have a minimum volume of _____ ml.

    a. 250
    b. 450
    c. 750
    d. 1000

35. A medication with positive inotropic effects is one that:

    a. increases heart rate
    b. increases myocardial contractility
    c. reduces myocardial oxygen consumption
    d. slows the rate of conduction through the AV node

36. For the unconscious, apneic and pulseless child in ventricular fibrillation, the initial amount of energy delivered is:

    a. 2 joules/kg, synchronized
    b. 4 joules/kg, synchronized
    c. 2 joules/kg, unsynchronized
    d. 4 joules/kg, unsynchronized

37. The maximum total dose of atropine is:

    a. 0.1 mg in a child, 0.5 mg in an adolescent
    b. 0.5 mg in a child, 1.0 mg in an adolescent
    c. 1.0 mg in a child, 2.0 mg in an adolescent
    d. 2.0 mg in a child, 3.0 mg in an adolescent

38. Tachycardia is best defined as:

    a. a heart rate greater than 100 beats per minute
    b. a heart rate greater than 200 beats per minute
    c. faster than the upper range of normal for age
    d. slower than the lower range of normal for age

39. The minimum recommended oxygen flow rate to be used with a self-inflating bag is:

    a. 3-5 liters/minute
    b. 5-8 liters/minute
    c. 8-10 liters/minute
    d. 10-15 liters/minute

40. You are asked to examine a 20-month old child with difficulty breathing. Mom states the child has had a runny nose and mild fever for the past two days. The child is crying and obvious stridor is noted. Examination of the child reveals a respiratory rate of 40 with equal chest rise and clear bilateral breath sounds. The child is pink, capillary refill is < 2 seconds, peripheral pulses are strong and regular, the skin is warm and dry. The heart rate is 110 beats/minute, temperature 100.4-degrees.

    Is this child in respiratory failure or shock? _____

41. Describe your initial management priorities in the treatment of this child.

_____

_____

42. A seven year old victim of a submersion incident is pulseless and apneic. CPR is in progress. The cardiac monitor displays the rhythm below. Attempts to establish intravenous access have proved unsuccessful.

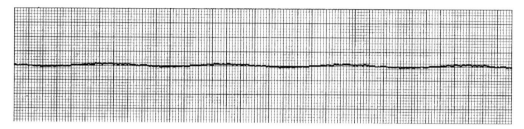

Figure 9-3.

The rhythm shown is: _____.

43. The first medication that should be administered in this situation is:

     a. atropine
     b. lidocaine
     c. dopamine
     d. epinephrine

44. Intravenous access has not been established. The medication mentioned in the previous question should be administered:

     a. endotracheally
     b. subcutaneously
     c. by intraosseous infusion
     d. by intramuscular injection

45. Early shock is diagnosed by evaluation of:

     1. heart rate
     2. presence and strength of peripheral pulses
     3. adequacy of end-organ perfusion

     a. 1, 2
     b. 1, 3
     c. 2, 3
     d. 1, 2, 3

46. Describe the ECG characteristics of sinus tachycardia.

    Rate: _____

    Rhythm: _____

    P waves: _____

    QRS: _____

    T waves: _____

47. A neonate is an infant:
    a. less than one week of age
    b. less than one month of age
    c. less than six months of age
    d. less than twelve months of age

48. Atropine is available in prefilled syringes containing 1 mg/ 10 ml (0.1 mg/ml). The correct initial dose of atropine administered to a 20-kg child, in milligrams and milliliters, would be:
    a. 0.1 mg, 1 ml
    b. 0.2 mg, 2 ml
    c. 0.4 mg, 4 ml
    d. 0.5 mg, 5 ml

49. Which of the following statements is **INCORRECT** regarding umbilical cannulation?
    a. the lumen of the umbilical vein is larger than that of the umbilical artery
    b. complications of this procedure include embolism, portal vein thrombosis and infection
    c. a 5F umbilical catheter is inserted into the vessel so the tip is just below the skin and there is free flow of blood
    d. the umbilical artery is recognized as a thin-walled single vessel in contrast to the umbilical veins that are paired, thicker walled and often constricted

50. Which of the following statements regarding intraosseous cannulation is **INCORRECT?**
    a. the intraosseous site is not a site of first choice for vascular access.
    b. medications administered via this route should be followed with a fluid flush to facilitate delivery into the central circulation
    c. intraosseous cannulation is a temporary measure, another form of vascular access should be sought once the child's condition is stabilized
    d. intraosseous cannulation is indicated in the child 12 years of age or younger when reliable venous access cannot be obtained within three attempts or 90 seconds, whichever comes first

POSTTEST ANSWERS

QUESTION	ANSWER	RATIONALE	STUDY GUIDE REFERENCE	PALS PAGE REFERENCE
1	D	Catheter-fragment embolism, sepsis, air embolism and pulmonary thromboembolism are systemic complications of intravascular access. Phlebitis, hematoma formation, and cellulitis are examples of local complications.	117	5-7
2	A	Stridor is a high-pitched inspiratory sound associated with upper airway obstruction.	49	2-3
3		The rhythm displayed is ventricular fibrillation.	160	N/A
4	A	The infant should be defibrillated up to three times if needed with 2 j/kg, 4 j/kg, 4 j/kg. Attempts to obtain IV or intraosseous access should be made but should not delay defibrillation.	169	7-8
5	B	Naloxone (Narcan) is a narcotic antagonist.	201	6-9
6	C	Signs of respiratory failure include cyanosis, diminished breath sounds, decreased level of consciousness or response to pain, poor skeletal muscle tone, and inadequate respiratory rate, effort or chest excursion	44	2-2
7	A	Oxygen-powered breathing devices are not recommended for pediatric use because tidal volume is difficult to control and high airway pressure may develop, producing gastric distention (with mask ventilation) or tension pneumothorax.	98	4-18
8	D	Motor vehicle-related trauma accounts for nearly 1/2 of all pediatric injuries and deaths.	20	3-2

9	C	Primary causes of circulatory failure in children include: 1. Hypovolemic (loss of vascular volume) - fluid loss (burns, vomiting, diarrhea), blood loss due to trauma 2. Distributive (loss of peripheral vascular resistance) - sepsis, anaphylaxis, spinal cord injury 3. Cardiogenic (cardiac failure) - congenital heart disease, heart rate abnormalities, cardiomyopathy Epiglottitis and foreign-body airway obstruction are precipitating causes of respiratory distress and failure.	46	2-4
10	D	An endotracheal intubation attempt should take no longer than 30 seconds. The heart rate should be monitored during the procedure. If bradycardia occurs or the child's color or perfusion deteriorates, the intubation attempt should be interrupted and the patient ventilated with a bag-mask device and supplemental oxygen.	103-106	4-14
11	A	Crystalloid solutions are inexpensive, readily available and free from allergic reactions. Colloid solutions are expensive, have a short shelf-life, are more likely to cause adverse reactions and are efficient in rapidly expanding the intravascular compartment.	139-140	6-1
12	C	Cessation of ventilation and circulation results in a mixed respiratory and metabolic **acidosis.**		6-3
13	A	VF is seen in less than 10% of pediatric cardiac arrests. When VF is present, a search for a metabolic abnormality, hypothermia or drug toxicity should be made.	160, 169	7-8
14	B	Lidocaine, epinephrine, atropine and naloxone may be administered IV, ET and IO. Sodium bicarbonate cannot be administered endotracheally. Dopamine is administered as a continuous infusion; it cannot be administered endotracheally.	98, 141	6-5

15	D	Bretylium is a ventricular antidysrhythmic that may be beneficial in the treatment of refractory VF or pulseless VT.	147	7-6
16	C	Complications of central venous cannulation include infection, air embolism, pneumothorax, hemothorax, hemorrhage, cardiac tamponade and catheter-fragment embolism.	120	5-7
17	B	Epinephrine increases heart rate, myocardial contractility, automaticity, systemic vascular resistance and myocardial oxygen requirements.	143	6-6
18		Cardiac output = stroke volume x heart rate. Very rapid rates result in decreased ventricular filling time, reducing stroke volume and, ultimately, cardiac output. (High heart rate x low stroke volume = low cardiac output)	157	7-3
19	A	Verapamil should not be used in infants because cardiac arrest has been reported following its administration (Class III - not indicated, may be harmful). Its use is discouraged in children since it may cause hypotension and myocardial depression.	145	7-5
20		Ventricular Tachycardia Rate: 120-400 beats/minute Rhythm: Essentially regular P waves: Usually not seen; if present, they have no set relationship to the QRS's appearing between the QRS complexes at a rate different from that of the VT QRS: > 0.08 sec (wide); may be difficult to differentiate between the QRS and the T wave T waves: Usually opposite in polarity to the QRS	158	7-5
21	B	The recommended endotracheal tube size for a six year old is 5.5 mm I.D. Formula: [Age (years)/4]+4 or 16 + patient's age (years)/4. Either formula can be used to determine size.	99	4-15

22	A	Self-inflating bags have an intake valve thatallows rapid reinflation of the bag. This valve results in dilution of the oxygen in the bag with room air. In order to deliver high concentrations of oxygen with this device, an oxygen reservoir must be attached.	93	4-11
23	B	Sodium bicarbonate is hyperosmolar, sclerosing to small veins and produces a chemical burn if extravasation occurs. Sodium bicarbonate is not administered endotracheally. Calcium may result in severe dysrhythmias in patients on digitalis.	144	6-8, 6-11
24		a. Weight = 8 + (years x 2) = 14 kg b. ET size = [years/4]+4 = 4.5 mm c. Systolic BP=70 + (2 x years) = 76 d. Heart rate = 80-110 e. Respiratory rate = 22-34	48, 55, 54, 99	2-5, 4-14
25		The inverted pyramid shows the a pproximate relative frequencies of neonatal resuscitation efforts. Most neonates respond to simple resuscitative measures.	188	9-1
26	A	The compression-ventilation ratio is 3:1 in the neonate.	199	9-6
27		The infant is showing signs of cardiopulmonary failure. Place the infant on high flow oxygen and attempt to establish IV access. Place the infant on a cardiac monitor and pulse oximetry.	64	2-7
28		a. The rhythm is fast with a ventricular rate greater than 200 beats/minute (recorded heart rate is 292 beats/min). The QRS is narrow and regular. This rhythm is supraventricular tachycardia. b. This infant is clearly unstable as evidenced by: delayed capillary refill, cyanosis, lethargy, cool extremities and absence of palpable distal pulses.	168	7-4

29	B	Since an IV is already in place, adenosine may be administered before synchronized countershock. If there is no effect, the dose may be doubled. If synchronized countershock is performed, the initial energy used is 0.5 joules/kg. Verapamil is not recommended for use in children. Defibrillation is used for VF and pulse-less ventricular tachycardia. Lidocaine is indicated for ventricular rhythms. This rhythm (narrow QRS) is supraventricular in origin.	168	7-4, 7-5
30		When the baby's head is delivered (before the shoulders), suction the nose, mouth and pharynx with a 12F or larger suction catheter. Remove residual meconium with suction when the infant has been placed on a radiant warmer and before drying by visualizing the pharynx with a laryngoscope. Follow with intubation of the trachea and suctioning of the lower airway. This infant should not be stimulated or bagged before clearing the airway of the thick meconium.	202-203	9-8
31		This infant is showing signs of early (compensated) shock. The history and clinical presentation are consistent with moderate dehydration.	61, 68	2-4, 2-8
32		Administer high flow oxygen and establish vascular access. Place the infant on a cardiac monitor and pulse oximetry. When vascular access is obtained, administer a 20 ml/kg bolus of normal saline or Ringer's lactate (in < 20 minutes). Reassess after the bolus has been administered and give additional fluids based on the infant's response to treatment.	64	2-7, 6-2
33	C	Dopamine is used in the treatment of circulatory shock following resuscitation or when shock is unresponsive to fluid administration (Class I - definitely helpful). The recommended dosage range is 2-20 mcg/kg/min. The half-life of dopamine is short, thus it must be administered by continuous infusion.	148	6-12

34	B	Neonatal-size (250 ml) ventilation bags may be inadequate to support effective tidal volume and the longer inspiratory times required by full-term neonates and infants. The minimum recommended volume for resuscitation bags used for ventilation of full-term neonates, infants and children is 450 ml.	94	9-6
35	B	Inotrope refers to myocardial contractility. A drug that is a positive inotrope increases myocardial contractility (such as dopamine, epinephrine). A drug that is a negative inotrope decreases myocardial contractility (such as verapamil).	139	N/A
36	C	Defibrillation (unsynchronized countershock) is indicated in VF or pulseless ventricular tachycardia. The first 3 defibrillation attempts should be delivered in rapid succession. The recommended initial energy is 2 joules/kg followed with 4 joules/kg and again with 4 joules/kg.	169	7-9
37	C	The recommended dose of atropine is 0.02 mg/kg with a minimum dose of 0.1 mg and a maximum single dose of 0.5 mg in a child and 1.0 mg in an adolescent. The dose may be repeated in five minutes to a maximum total dose of 1.0 mg in a child and 2.0 mg in an adolescent.	146	6-9, 6-15
38	C	Tachycardia is best defined as a rate faster than the upper range of normal for age.	155	7-3
39	D	An oxygen flow rate of at least 10-15 liters/minute is necessary to maintain an adequate oxygen volume in the reservoir of a self-inflating pediatric bag.	95	4-12
40		This child is exhibiting signs of potential respiratory failure. The child's age, clinical signs and history are consistent with croup.	44, 66	2-2
41		Administer supplemental oxygen in a nonthreatening manner and allow the child to assume a position of comfort (for example, allow mom to hold while administering blow-by O2). Maintain body temperature, give nothing by mouth and reassess frequently.	52	2-7

42		The rhythm shown is asystole. Confirm the rhythm in another lead, continue CPR, secure the airway with an endotracheal tube and hyperventilate with 100% oxygen.	160, 170	7-9
43	D	The first medication administered in the management of asystole is epinephrine.	170	7-9
44	A	The child should be intubated and epinephrine administered endotracheally. Intraosseous access is recommended for children six years of age or younger.	119	7-9
45	D	Early shock is diagnosed by evaluation of heart rate, presence and volume (strength) of peripheral pulses, and adequacy of end-organ perfusion. Sustained sinus tachycardia may be an early sign of cardiovascular compromise.	55	2-4
46		Sinus Tachycardia Rate: Faster than upper limit of normal for age, usually less than 200 beats/minute Rhythm: Usually regular but may vary P waves: Upright in Lead II, if discernible QRS: Within normal limits (narrow)	156-157	7-3
47	B	The term "neonate" is used to describe an infant less than 1 month of age.	187	N/A
48	C	The recommended initial dose of atropine is 0.02 mg/kg. Atropine is supplied as 1 mg/10 ml. The initial dose (in milligrams) to be administered to a 20-kg child is 0.4 mg. This would equal 4 ml of the supplied solution.	146	6-9, 6-15
49	D	The umbilical vein is recognized as a thin-walled single vessel in contrast to the umbilical arteries which are paired, thicker walled and often constricted.	199-200	9-7
50	D	Intraosseous cannulation is indicated in the child six years of age or younger when reliable venous access cannot be obtained within three attempts or 90 seconds, whichever comes first.	119, 125	5-2

Index